THE MEDICAL RACKET

Other Books by Martin L. Gross

Nonfiction

THE END OF SANITY
Social and Cultural Madness in America

THE GOVERNMENT RACKET
Washington Waste From A to Z

A CALL FOR REVOLUTION
How Washington Is Strangling America

THE POLITICAL RACKET
Deceit, Self-Interest and Corruption in American Politics

THE TAX RACKET

THE PSYCHOLOGICAL SOCIETY

THE BRAIN WATCHERS

THE DOCTORS

Fiction

MAN OF DESTINY

THE MEDICAL RACKET

How Doctors, HMOs, and Hospitals Are Failing the American Patient

MARTIN L. GROSS

AVON BOOKS 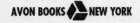 NEW YORK

AVON BOOKS, INC.
1350 Avenue of the Americas
New York, New York 10019

Library of Congress Cataloging in Publication Data:

Gross, Martin L. (Martin Louis), 1935–
    The medical racket : how doctors, HMOs, and hospitals are failing the American
patient / Martin L. Gross.
        p.   cm.
    Includes bibliographical references and index.
    1. Medical care—Corrupt practices—United States. 2. Medical errors—United
States. I. Title.
RA395.A3G75 1998   98-25668
362.1'0973—dc21   CIP

First Avon Books Trade Paperback Printing: November 1998

AVON TRADEMARK REG. U.S. PAT. OFF. AND IN OTHER COUNTRIES, MARCA REGISTRADA, HECHO
EN U.S.A.

Printed in the U.S.A.

OPM   10 9 8 7 6 5 4 3 2

Contents

v

                The Knife and You

CHAPTER VI: THE MAKING OF A MODERN   191
                DOCTOR
                Coddling the Medical School
                Student: Easy In, Easy Through

CHAPTER VII: MEDICAL ECONOMICS AND   213
                THE AMERICAN DOCTOR
                Business Before Healing

CHAPTER VIII: A PLAN FOR TOMORROW   230
                How to Reform Medicine
                and Eliminate the Chaos

                Notes and Bibliography   243

                Index   262

                About the Author   278

THE MEDICAL RACKET

Introduction

Nothing touches the human psyche more powerfully than concerns over sickness and health, the landmarks of life and death.

The fear of sickness has always been a compulsive one among us humans. For centuries we have believed that profound help was available from physicians, even though that belief rested more on faith and superstition than on science.

Hundreds of years ago many in Western nations lived as long, or longer, than today. Jefferson survived into his mid-eighties. John Adams died when he was ninety. In fact, the first ten American presidents lived to an average of seventy-eight years, a full decade longer than later leaders, not counting those who were assassinated.

That longevity, of course, did not include many millions of their day who failed to survive into old age, taken

1

prematurely by such scourges as diphtheria, cholera, smallpox, the death of mothers and infants in childbirth, and infections and diseases that have since then been partially conquered by medical science.

But it wasn't until World War II, medical historian Arthur K. Shapiro reminded us, that there was a net benefit from the profession of medicine. Prior to that, most gains were actually the result of the improved lifestyle of the emerging middle class, good sanitation, and the placebo effect, which seems to mobilize the body's defenses without intervention. Medicine itself was still basically a shaman worship of sorts. Some lives were saved, others eased, but that small benefit was wiped out by sickness and death from iatrogenic, or doctor-caused, disease.

Now, a half century later, there finally *is* a measurable benefit to the public from the profession—the saving and extending of lives. Doctors, who have always been held in high esteem, even when their medical armamentarium was negligible, have benefited along with their patients. Their incomes and prestige are now enormous, greater even than during the less scientific era when doctors expertly consoled and postured, rather than healed.

Clinical medicine, the day-to-day treatment of patients, is better today than in 1967, when I wrote *The Doctors*, a critical analysis of the profession. In a long editorial, the American Medical Association attacked my numerous recommendations, only to try—after a sudden reformation—to implement most of them.

But did they finally succeed? Is the current medical profession blameless, efficient, dedicated, educated, honest, and responsive to the needs of the community overall?

Chaos Rules

Hardly. The system has never before been as unstable, with chaos ruling the medical arena, with no one sure what the future will hold in terms of a system of quality care that people can afford.

Some of the failings are old unresolved ones. There are also dozens of new problems and doctor failings, including distortions in medical care delivery unimaginable just thirty years ago. The intrusion of HMOs into the doctor's office and our hospitals in the name of economy presents a threat whose full dimensions we are only beginning to understand.

Economic problems that dogged us are now exaggerated, resulting in greater selfishness and exploitation by the profession, and an annual cost of medicine that exceeds any emperor's ransom and our ability to pay for it.

Training and selection of doctors, which had greatly progressed in the 1970s and 1980s, has retrogressed in many ways, creating more incompetent practitioners than ever before.

Clinical care, which was improving, is now being subject to new rules, systems, and regulations from the outside, which punish both good medicine and good doctors. Surgery is still too often unnecessary. Medical fraud, always a small problem, has become near epidemic. American hospitals are adrift, struggling against empty beds, fierce competition, and massive confusion.

Chilling New Crisis

American medicine today is in an economic, personal, and governmental crisis. Factors other than good health care—increasing control by insurers, the conflict between science and profit—are all working against the goal of ideal medicine.

In many ways, as we shall see, medicine is moving backward rather than forward even as new scientific advances are made daily.

We shall look beyond the taboos of the profession to closely examine physicians, hospitals, insurers, and medical colleges and their students, after which we will offer reasoned suggestions on how to solve the many problems. In a burst of optimism, we will try to redesign much of the conventional system of medical care in America at the turn of the new century.

From out of the current chaos, it is possible that a new, better era for the American patient may yet emerge.

Chapter 1

The HMO Revolution

They Profit, You Suffer

In California, a father became troubled when he learned that his nine-year-old daughter had a rare kidney cancer called a "Wilm's Tumor."

Seeking the best care possible for the child, he was pleased that his HMO covered the Lucile Packard Children's Hospital in Palo Alto. The hospital had a pediatric surgeon experienced in removing just such a tumor.

The operation was a success and the happy parent was in the intensive care unit with his daughter when he received a call from the "utilization nurse" of the HMO. "The bill is fifty thousand dollars," she told the father, "but you didn't get preapproval, so we're not going to pay you."

Though the surgeon and hospital were ostensibly included in his HMO plan, a technicality had left him out in the fiscal cold. His daughter's pediatric surgeon was in

5

the HMO, but he wasn't in their medical subgroup and therefore not covered, according to the HMO. The father was told that he should have used a urologist in his subgroup—an adult surgeon with no experience in this type of rare tumor.

The shocked and angered parent paid the bill but then took the HMO into arbitration. After a year, he got his money back, but the HMO refused to pay his heavy legal bills. He complained to the California Department of Corporations, which fined the HMO a half-million dollars.

This parent was finally vindicated, having only a temporary loss of money. But in this case, as in many, the once-vaunted HMOs, which were to cure all of medicine's problems, leave a lot to be desired. Not only are they not a true remedy, but they have actually worsened the medical situation with their overconcern with bottom-line profit at the expense of the best possible care.

Denial of Needed Care

In Kansas City a distraught soccer mom raced her boy to the emergency room of St. Luke's, the nearest hospital. He had broken his leg, and she waited nervously as the doctor started an IV (intravenous) to give him pain medication before he set the bone. The mother left for a moment to call the HMO that handles her insurance.

"Stop!" the mother shouted to the emergency room doctor when she returned. She explained that her son could not be treated there. She would have to go to a hospital that was four miles away that was covered by her plan.

The child was given an oral pain killer, a splint, and ice bag, and the parent had to seek "insured" care elsewhere.

The stories of medical treatment denied to patients by HMOs because they cost too much, or because the providers were out of their geographic area, or because a doctor or hospital wasn't part of their plan, are endless. Just as fee-for-service medicine can be dogged by expensive overtreatment and physician greed, so the managed care business has too often become a slave to irrational undertreatment.

For many HMOs, a penny saved on medical care is a penny more for the HMO executives and stockholders, a curious distortion of the Hippocratic Oath.

HMOs seem to enjoy denying medical care to subscribers. Why shouldn't they? Premiums from HMOs and other insurers run to $325 billion a year, and every operation and lab test refused means they get to keep more money in their pocket.

The truth of this attitude is sworn to by witnesses on the inside. One of these is Dr. Lina Peeno, head of the ethics committee at the University of Louisville Hospital, who spent six years working for health insurers—denying claims. "I naively thought that what they wanted was a physician who would bring medical knowledge to those claims that were open to interpretation," she explains. "What I found out was that the goal was to avoid paying for as much as possible."

The two major excuses insurers employ are that a treatment is "not medically necessary," or in the case of HMOs, they use obscure details to bounce claims. "If somebody doesn't follow the dots exactly right," adds Dr. Peeno, "then you can say, 'Well, sorry, you did not follow the rules'; I knew as a medical director that very few people appealed claims."

The HMOs often require preapproval for any serious expenditure, then use the power of 20–20 hindsight to turn down claims later on. If a patient fears he's suffering a heart attack, but it turns out to be only gastritis, those claims, Dr. Peeno says, are denied "right and left."

This HMO trick can be widespread. In Jefferson City, Missouri, a patient was told by her doctor that she needed a laparoscopy. Hewing to the requirement for preapproval, she notified her HMO and the procedure was done. But when she submitted her claim to the HMO, she was told she had not submitted her claim in time. She appealed, sending in the hospital's verification of precertification.

Once again, her legitimate claim was denied by the HMO, this time with a new excuse. Now they said that the procedure was not medically necessary. Finally, in desperation, she contacted the Missouri Department of Insurance (good advice for all frustrated patients), who decided she was correct. They instructed the HMO to pay her $4,500.

Dr. Michael E. DeBakey, the medical giant who pioneered the heart bypass operation and recently advised Russian doctors on the treatment of President Yeltsin, is disgusted with how HMOs limit freedom of choice, in effect trading health and lives for dollars—the opposite of the true medical goal.

He describes a case in which a woman came to see him at the DeBakey Heart Center in Houston. She had, he reports, "a dissecting aneurysm of the aorta, a type of heart disease that is rapidly fatal when not treated by the corrective operation" that he devised.

The woman, who belonged to an HMO, had been told that they would not approve the operation. A doctor relative put her in touch with Dr. DeBakey, who volunteered to do the surgery without charge. But the HMO would not approve the hospital costs, which would be substantial.

"Only after another family member—a lawyer this time—kicked up a fuss did the HMO grant the woman the chance to live by approving her hospitalization costs," DeBakey explains. "This is a lucid example of how patients become the victims of cost containment through restrictions on their freedom of choice."

Former U.S. Surgeon General C. Everett Koop concurs. "Whatever its flaws, traditional fee-for-service medicine always allowed physicians to act as advocates for their patients. HMOs cannot assure us that physicians will, in every instance, put their patients' interests first."

The failure of HMOs is especially apparent in situations like the one described by Dr. DeBakey, where expert help is needed in complex cases and is not available from the HMO.

A 54-year-old woman in New York lost her regular insurance when her employer switched to an HMO. When she was later diagnosed with intestinal cancer, an HMO surgeon removed the tumor. But when the cancer spread to her liver, the doctor and a cancer specialist from the HMO recommended she see a New Jersey surgeon who specialized in liver tumors. But the HMO refused to pay for the treatment. The renowned subspecialist was not in their "network." After months of hassle, they finally agreed to the treatment, but it was too late.

The HMO "Gatekeeper"

That lack of freedom is especially important when it comes to specialists, the star of American medicine. Men like DeBakey collectively offer the world's best clinical care. These doctors, in some forty specialties—from pediatric surgery to oncology—are fully available to fee-for-service patients, to most on Medicare, but not to many HMO subscribers.

Despite the near impossibility of properly caring for a serious ailment without a specialist, it is not always possible to see one in the world of HMO medicine. The HMO family, or "primary," doctor makes the decisions about patient care and can shut out the specialist when he wants.

The goal of this "gatekeeper," as he is called, is as often financial as medical. One of his jobs is to save money for the group, and specialists cost money. In fact, in some HMOs, part of the money saved by limiting specialist referrals may, as we shall see, end up right in the primary doctor's pocket.

There are numerous stories of seriously ill people who are denied the services of a specialist. It is, prima facie, a violation of medical ethics, yet is commonplace in HMOs, a form of medical philosophy almost exclusively based on cutting costs.

- A female family doctor severely injured her back in a plane crash and became paralyzed in the lower half of her body. Later on, when she returned to school to retrain as a psychiatrist, she was enrolled in the college's HMO.

She visited her primary doctor and asked to see a specialist in rehabilitation medicine. As a physician, she knew she should have a kidney test, for instance, because the catheter she was using for urination was susceptible to infection. But she says her "gatekeeper" turned down her request.

A month later she developed a pressure sore on her buttocks that opened and drained pus. But her primary doctor again refused to refer her to a specialist. Finally, she needed surgery to remove a portion of her buttocks and required three months in a nursing home. The result was that she had to drop out of school and hasn't worked since.

- In San Diego, a health consultant who had been under a three-year treatment with a specialist for allergy shots switched to PacifiCare because it was provided by his wife's employer. His new primary physician at the HMO decided to stop the treatment, which was in its final year. Soon after, his painful sinus infections returned, forcing the patient into bed. But this consumer didn't take it lying down. He complained to the state; to the National Committee of Quality Assurance, which accredits the HMOs; to the American Medical Association; and even to the White House.

Finally, PacifiCare reversed their position and sent him to an allergist. "They wear the patient out with all the administrative work," the patient said. The HMO answer inadvertently revealed the disturbing, destructive aspect of this relatively new type of medicine: "He is used to operating in the old fee-for-service medicine, where he went to a doctor whenever he wanted to see the doctor. With an HMO it's different."

That's for sure. The unfortunate result can come in every possible combination of damage, from denied or not extended medical care.

- In Manhattan, Congressman Jerrold Nadler described the sad HMO experience of his mother-in-law. Despite her history of breast cancer, the HMO doctor refused to order a CAT scan. By the time she finally had the test, the recurring cancer was too widespread to treat.
- In Brooklyn, an HMO wanted to send a patient's newborn triplets home from the hospital's neonatal unit even though his doctor said they might need special care for another month or more.
- Also in New York City, a union-based HMO refused to pay for the chemotherapy treatment of a woman member with breast cancer. Her internist, Dr. Bernard Kruger, tried to reach the union president, but his calls were never returned. The doctor was forced to appeal to the manufacturer, who contributed the needed chemotherapy drugs free of charge.

The HMOs' Dangerous Delays

When Americans think of bad medicine, Britain's National Health Service comes to mind, mainly because of endless bureaucracy and delays. Some people there wait for over a year for elective surgery.

It hasn't yet reached that stage in the American HMO "revolution," but the new system is already suffering from bureaucratic arthritis.

Take the example of a California housewife who reported disquieting symptoms to her HMO doctor, which could possibly have represented ovarian cancer. The HMO first gave approval for diagnostic surgery, which can be an expensive procedure. They went so far as to prep her for the operation while she waited at the hospital. Then, suddenly, the HMO withdrew permission for the surgery.

She waited and waited, while the HMO continued to delay the operation. Finally, ten months after her first visit she had the diagnostic surgery. It turned out that she did indeed have a cancerous growth on her ovary, which was finally removed.

"They had no regard for my life, safety, or health," she says of the bureaucracy at Health Net, California's second largest HMO.

Judging by stories from this and other disgruntled HMO subscribers, delays in treatment are quite common in some HMOs. One California HMO patient learned that he had prostate cancer and needed surgery. He waited and waited, and not until three months later was he operated on. Why? Because the medical group chosen by his HMO didn't have enough urologists to handle the traffic.

In another case, a primary care doctor in California tells of a patient who had rectal bleeding and needed a routine colonoscopy. But ten days passed, with still more bleeding, until the doctor received "authorization" for the procedure.

Some of these bureaucratic delays can be quite frustrating for patients and physicians. When a doctor prescribed a drug not on the HMO's "formulary"—a list of acceptable pharmaceuticals—the patient had to wait three months and badger the HMO with fifteen phone calls before she received permission to receive it. There are some critics who speculate that the delay is a method of keeping the patient at bay in the hope that she will finally give up—saving money for the "managed care" operation.

One of the most grievous items in the HMO bag of tricks is to force doctors to prescribe cheaper drugs, even if they're not as effective as the ones he'd like to give his patients.

The HMOs have hired firms called "pharmaceutical benefit managers," or PBMs, whose job is to lean on doctors and druggists to prescribe favored pharmaceuticals, sometimes offering pharmacists cash ($12 per prescription) if he successfully switches to a favored substitute from what the doctor ordered. Often the substitute is made by a drug company of which the PBM is a subsidiary.

New York City Public Advocate Mark Green reports that his investigation into this legal scam shows that substitute drugs (not generic, which are the same formula) are often chemically different and less effective medically, and sometimes even dangerous.

Each HMO strives to get their doctors to stick to the formulary. "If the physician displays a tendency to prescribe nonpreferred drugs," the report quotes the pharmacy director at Aetna, "he either gets a letter or a phone call and sometimes a nurse's visit to educate and inform him about the plan's preferred drugs and to ensure compliance with them."

Doctors who go along with this nonsense, and there are many who do, should be aware that they are violating the Hippocratic Oath.

And yet, surprisingly, the overwhelming majority of subscribers are happy with their HMOs. Or perhaps it is not so surprising. Most people are healthy and do not require complex treatment. When it comes to routine cases, the "primary" physician is usually quite sufficient to the challenge, especially since the majority of ailments are self-corrective over time.

That's the theoretical failure of the HMO scheme. The economics of the system is based on taking in premiums from the healthy and withholding as much care from the sick as possible, short of triggering a patient, or political, revolution against the situation.

What of the truly sick? What do they think of their HMOs? A poll of patient satisfaction shows that HMO popularity decreases among the old, the chronically ill, and those who need special attention. Of those who described their health as "poor," twice as many HMO patients were dissatisfied with their care as were patients in fee-for-service.

A study by Dr. John Ware of the New England Medical Center, published in *JAMA*, showed that a *majority* of elderly patients in HMOs reported a decline in health over a four-year period as against only 28 percent in fee-for-service plans.

Another study, conducted by researchers at the Virginia Commonwealth University, and also published in *JAMA*, showed that aged stroke victim subscribers to an HMO are more likely to be shipped off to a nursing home than to a more expensive but medically superior rehabilitation center—in the ratio of 42 to 28 percent.

Desperation in the Emergency Room

One strong bone of contention is that HMOs interfere with what was once considered standard medical care. This is especially true when a subscriber comes into an emergency room in desperate need.

The *Los Angeles Times* reported on the case of a pregnant woman who arrived in the Anaheim Memorial Hospital in the throes of a miscarriage. She was in extreme pain and bleeding profusely. A staff member gave her a quick exam and called her HMO, Tower Health, for insurance approval of the treatment. It took Tower two and a half hours to call back, and they still didn't grant approval. For six hours afterward, the physicians insist, they and Tower argued over who was responsible for the cost of the woman's treatment.

The conflict between HMOs and emergency rooms is in-built and loaded against the patient. This is a nationwide problem, which is only now being examined in some states. Unlike most other patients—those insured by Medicare, Medicaid, or private insurance, who can go to *any* emergency room and get unquestioned treatment at any time—HMO subscribers are often restricted to plan-approved emergency rooms.

This, of course, negates the whole concept of the "open door" emergency medicine that is supposed to be available to anyone anywhere in America at any time. The HMO/emergency room setup seems, at the very least, like a violation of medical ethics, and perhaps worse.

Denying Needed Care

One of the gravest drawbacks of HMOs is that the newest advances in medicine are often denied to subscribers because of their cost. The case of a sixteen-year-old boy, an honor student in suburban New Jersey who suffered from inadequate growth, was reported in the New York *Post*. He was only five-one, even though both his parents were taller than average. He also suffered from delayed puberty, and still had the squeaky voice of a child. The HMO approved a visit to an endocrinologist, who discovered that the young man had a growth hormone deficiency. Not enough of the substance was being produced by his pituitary gland.

The endocrinologist believed that with daily injections of a drug called Protropin, three times a day for three years, he was expected to grow to a height of five-eleven. The problem was the cost of the shots: $50,000 a year, which his parents couldn't afford.

The request to the HMO that they cover the treatment was rejected. The treatment, the HMO said, was not covered by their policy. Months went by, along with letters and pleas from the parents and the endocrinologist. But the HMO refused to budge. Finally, the *Post* got involved and approached the HMO. Six days later the treatment was approved. The family's only cost was their maximum deductible of $4,200 a year, a lot better than the impossible $50,000 annual price.

If the newest high-tech medical procedures, which are often expensive, are denied to HMO patients, the whole managed care movement may become a shaky, unacceptable alternative to fee-for-service medicine. This despite the supposed savings in cost, which may prove to be temporary in any case, as we shall see. As expensive as the older system may have been, it seldom denied medical care to ailing patients, especially when it was a matter of life or death.

In most states, all an HMO patient can do when denied treatment is to appeal back to the HMO—a highly unsatisfactory situation. However, California and New Jersey have taken the lead and set up arbitration panels to which HMO subscribers can take their complaints about denied treatment. Other states are contemplating the same.

The problem is that, in New Jersey for example, the panel's decisions are non-binding. However, says the state's health commissioner, he expects the HMOs to voluntarily follow the recommendations "99 percent" of the time.

They Call It "Experimental"

The refusal to pay for modern treatments usually available at university teaching hospitals is cleverly handled by the HMO by labeling it "experimental," the word managed care bureaucrats use when they mean "expensive."

In advanced stages of cancer, for instance, often the last hope of survival is a technique known as "bone marrow transplant." In this procedure, the physicians take out a portion of the bone marrow *before* the patient undergoes chemotherapy. Once collected outside the body, the cancer cells in the removed marrow are destroyed. After the patient is treated with chemotherapy, the bone marrow is reinfused into the patient in the hope that it will grow new marrow that is not cancerous. (A similar treatment has also been developed using blood stem cells.)

This treatment is almost commonplace at facilities like Memorial Sloan-Kettering Hospital in New York, perhaps the nation's leading cancer center. But it is virtually impossible for subscribers of the HMOs, where money plays the dominant role in whether or not to grant such treatment.

In California, Nelene Fox, a woman in her forties, had metastatic breast cancer that did not yield to conventional chemotherapy. Her doctors recommended very high dose chemotherapy and a bone marrow transplant. Her HMO, Health Net, turned down the expensive treatment. Instead, she raised the money privately and underwent the transplant. Despite it, she died eight months later.

Following her death, her brother sued the HMO. The jury agreed that the HMO had acted in bad faith and awarded the Fox family $89 million, which was later negotiated downward. The *California Physician*, official organ of the California Medical Association, summed up the problem succinctly:

"The case highlighted a growing distrust by patients, not only of the health plans, but of physicians."

Betsy McCaughey Ross, then the lieutenant governor of New York, used the op-ed page of the *New York Times* to describe another such case.

John Crescenzo, a 44-year-old truck driver, paid $6,000 a year in premiums to Wellcare, an HMO. When he developed a large lump on his thigh, Wellcare doctors eventually diagnosed it as a sarcoma, a rare cancer. They tried surgery and chemotherapy, but it spread to his lungs.

Doctors agreed that his best chance for survival was a form of experimental chemotherapy at Memorial Sloan-Kettering Cancer Center, where a surgeon agreed to operate without charge.

But Wellcare turned down the hospitalization, then again denied treatment on appeal. To whom? Wellcare. As Ms. Ross says: "Your opponent is also your judge and jury."

An HMO on Trial

The whole question of how money shapes medical care at HMOs was tested in court in Dallas, Texas, in December 1997. The plaintiff's family charged that the local Kaiser Permanente Health Plan had contributed to the death of fifty-six-year-old Ronald Henderson because they were employing cost-cutting procedures at their clinic, where Henderson dropped dead of a heart attack.

The case was based more on general policy than on specific medical facts. In a way, it became a symbolic trial of HMOs and their cost-cutting techniques. Americans are increasingly skeptical of HMOs in that regard, as a recent poll showed. Fifty-five percent suspected that economics took priority over quality care among HMOs.

A "minitrial" was held before a summary jury—a short hearing that is not binding, but is a preview of what a full jury might decide. Kaiser Permanente claimed that the patient was an overweight smoker who didn't obey doctor's orders, which was why, they asserted, he died— and not because of their economic considerations.

The plaintiffs countered by offering evidence that the Kaiser operation in Texas was dominated by cost-cutting. One piece of evidence was a speech made by an associate medical director of the Permanente Medical Association of Texas at a managed care convention.

"The first thing that ever comes out of a Kaiser CEO now is what's the bottom line," he was quoted as saying. "I'm trained to do that now almost automatically."

According to a report in the *Dallas Morning News*, the medical director allegedly also said that doctors at Kaiser's Urgent Care Centers in North Texas were told not to talk to patients about hospitalization. Instead, they were told to call in another doctor. "We basically said [to] the UCC doctors, 'If you value your job, you won't say anything about hospitalization. All you'll say is, "I think you need further evaluation. . . ." ' "

Another piece of evidence that spoke to the issue of poorer medical care was a Texas Permanente plan that discussed ways to "agressively reduce costs," including cutting hospital expenses by *almost half* (forty-five percent) and reducing outpatient costs twenty percent.

Before the summary jury (which said they would have granted a $62 million judgment against Kaiser) could report back, the parties settled. The Henderson family was awarded $5.3 million, even though Kaiser didn't admit any blame.

Who was right? In a way, both. The economy moves may not have been *specifically* related to Mr. Henderson's death, but cost-cutting surely plays a large part in how patients are medically cared for by HMOs. The pressure to cut costs in the Kaiser operation in Fort Worth–Dallas, for instance, is quite strong. That HMO had a $42-million loss in 1997, following two prior years of losses.

Kaiser is one of the largest managed care plans in the nation, with almost nine million subscribers. What makes this case particularly interesting is that Kaiser often scores as number one in surveys of the nation's best HMOs. One reason is that they directly employ eight thousand physicians nationwide who work on salary, rather than being totally dependent on meager fees for each person covered. Kaiser also runs over three hundred clinics in the United States, and has a hospital chain of its own in California, Oregon, and Hawaii. However, in its recent moves to become competitive and to expend where they don't have their own facilities, quality may well be suffering.

HMO Secrets Kept from Patients

The HMO industry's drive to cut costs nationwide can be so intense that they don't even want patients to know that there are other good but possibly more expensive treatments out there that are not covered by their plan. It seems that a truly educated medical consumer can be an HMO's worst customer.

This was the case of a neurologist who had worked with a large HMO. She advised the mother of a brain-damaged man that a muscle biopsy could help diagnose the extent of his condition. To her dismay she discovered that her attempts to educate her patients were not appreciated by her HMO boss.

"I was told that it was a mistake to tell the patient

about a procedure before checking to see whether it was covered," she relates.

Dr. David Himmelstein, an associate professor of medicine at Harvard Medical School, has been in the forefront of exposing these "gag rules," subtle and otherwise. In essence, these rules warn doctors not to say anything to patients that might end up costing the HMO money.

The HMOs are not stupid. They generally do not spell it out explicitly. Instead, the participating doctor has to sign a clause in his HMO contract that states it *implicitly.* Dr. Himmelstein himself joined up with an HMO, U.S. Healthcare, which presented him with a contract. One clause read:

"Physicians shall agree not to take any action or make any communication which undermines or could undermine that confidence of enrollees, potential enrollees, their employers, their unions, or the public, in U.S. Healthcare or the quality of U.S. Healthcare coverage."

Dr. Himmelstein crossed out the offensive clause and then signed the contract, which was accepted anyway. (He has since left U.S. Healthcare, which has been merged with Aetna insurance.) But he is a singular exception. Other doctors sign on to this obligation, which runs counter to their Hippocratic Oath: that the patient be paramount in all of a doctor's activities.

Gag Rule Legislation

Several states have already passed legislation outlawing the offensive gag rule, and Washington has resolved to stop it in Medicare HMO plans, but the American Association of Health Plans, the HMO industry group, denies they even exist. They quote a study of the U.S. government General Accounting Office, which was asked by Congress to look into the matter.

The GAO reported back that they have not found any *explicit* "gag orders" to doctors in the contracts they examined. But they did leave room open, saying some physicians are wary about being inhibited by clauses that keep them from disparaging any aspect of the HMO's covered treatments. In addition, the GAO points out that some 150 HMOs did not reply. These could well have explicit gag rules.

The stress that HMOs put on secrecy is evident. They try, sometimes desperately, not to disclose their methods—which are the basis of their profit system. Susan Rosenfeld, former general counsel to Memorial Sloan-Kettering Cancer Center in New York, says that "HMOs don't like to give information to prospective patients."

This became quite clear when the *New York Times* profiled a large consulting firm that advises, through guidelines, which services HMOs should and should not pay for. One extreme example of callousness was a guideline suggesting that HMOs pay for cataract surgery in only one eye, even if the patient had dual cataracts. The rationale? He only needed to see out of one eye!

This horrendous money saver has since been rescinded.

The consultant wanted the HMO to pinch every medical penny by moving patients out of the hospital, as if on an assembly line. They recommended only a twelve-hour stay for mothers who had just given birth: two days for someone whose leg had been amputated above the knee; and only four days after a heart bypass operation.

Less Medicine, More Kickbacks

Another way for HMOs to squeeze out the last dollar of profit is to reward doctors for practicing inferior medicine.

How is that done? Simple. In many HMOs, if doctors make *less* use of medical facilities and treatments, they will receive *more* in their paycheck. In 1996 the following substantial bonuses—some might call it a "kickback"—were given to doctors in a large HMO plan:

- If a doctor—who in this case had 925 patients—made sure that his patients collectively averaged less than 178 days in the hospital in any given year, he would receive a substantial bonus of $24,756.

- If emergency room visits of his patients averaged less than eighty-four cents per patient in any given month—or $744 in all—he would receive a bonus of $453 for that month. But if costs rose above $1.64 a month per patient, he would receive nothing.
- Other large bonuses were awarded for cutting down the number of subscribers referred to specialists, obviously reducing the quality of care of the sickest patients. If specialist cost per patient averaged less than $14.49 per month, the doctor would receive a bonus of $1,323 for the month, or an additional $15,876 for the year. But if costs rose above $30.49 per patient, he would get nothing. (Other HMOs give doctors bonuses for cutting back on lab tests as well.)

In a saner medical world, these bonuses would, ipso facto, be considered unethical physician behavior. If employers and politicians had not been hypnotized by the HMO promise of lower costs, agreement to such antimedical ideas might well result in the suspension of medical licenses.

A Case of Castration Anxiety

Stories of HMOs saving dollars at the expense of good medical care can challenge one's credulity. A patient in Florida, a seventy-six-year-old former New Yorker, was diagnosed as having prostate cancer. He was treated with daily injections of Lupron, an antihormonal drug intended to stop the spread of the disease. The cost to his HMO was $350 a month. The amount was apparently so troubling to the HMO that two physicians at their Florida health center recommended that the patient be castrated instead!

When the patient protested that he didn't want to be

castrated, he was reminded that his medicine was expensive. Castration, he was told, would be more "cost effective" for the HMO.

Unlike many of the aged, who don't have the skill or energy to protest, this man went to the state health-care administrator, who ordered the HMO to continue the injections.

One of the basic ways that HMOs save money is their system of "capitation." A doctor will be given a set amount per year per patient to handle the medical care of perhaps five hundred patients. For that, he is supposed to provide "comprehensive medicine," including immunization and preventive medicine. *But in reality the capitation more often works as an incentive gimmick for the doctor to cut down the amount of quality care he performs or authorizes.*

Since he receives his money in advance, the less time he spends on his capitated patients, the more money the doctor makes.

The Fight Against Capitation

"Capitation is against the idea of good medical care, and is the incentive for the doctor to do less and keep the HMO happy," said Dr. Gordon A. Miller, an ophthalmologist in Salem, Oregon, when interviewed. "Under capitation, the doctor becomes an advocate of the HMO instead of for the patient."

Dr. Miller created Measure 35, which was a voter initiative attempt to reform HMOs in Oregon. It was designed to eliminate capitation and other HMO financial incentives that influence doctors to reduce the amount and cost of care. It was defeated two-to-one in the 1996 election.

"Why?" I asked Dr. Miller.

"For two reasons," he says. "First, there was a well-financed campaign by the managed care companies to defeat it. Secondly, they told the voters that if it passed, the employers might drop the HMOs entirely, and they would be without health insurance. The people decided that poor health care was better than none."

Dr. Miller outlined another doctor incentive common in HMO contracts:

"They call it 'withholding,' and it's a horrible method of persuading doctors to do less. What the HMOs do is hold back anywhere up to a third of the doctor's fee. They wait until the end of the year, when they tally the medical usage in a given pool of doctors—anywhere from ten to a hundred. I'm in a pool myself. If the doctors have cooperated by using less care—hospitals, specialists, lab tests—then the HMO releases all or part of the money back to the doctors at the year's end. But if the costs have run too high, the HMO keeps all of the withheld money. It's a very effective and very unethical way to run a medical system. It's really a form of medical blackmail."

Dr. Miller does business with a dozen HMOs, and as a specialist, receives fee-for-service renumeration. But he too is subject to the withholding gimmick.

"Sometimes they return some of the money," he said. "Last year they kept it all. The idea is to make me provide less medical care for my patients so that I'll get my money back. But I don't play ball with them. I do whatever is medically necessary. Now they plan to hold back twenty percent of my fee, and are threatening thirty percent. If they do that, I'll just drop all my HMOs. I'm lucky because most of my patients are seniors on Medicare, and I'm happy to accept the government fees. But some of my colleagues aren't so fortunate. They have to play ball or, as I say, sell out to the HMOs."

Dr. Miller tried to explain the complex flow of money in the HMO system in his area:

"The capitation method tries to make the 'primary' doctor, the 'gatekeeper,' into a partner in their insurance business. They have him risk part of his fee if he authorizes too much medical care. The HMO spreads his risk by placing him in a pool with other physicians. But he's still liable if things go wrong. In my state, not long ago, a group of eye doctors who accepted capitation actually went broke when one of the patients had to have five expensive surgeries to save her sight. Obviously, most doctor/gatekeepers are not going to risk that, so they watch every penny, which is just what the HMOs want. This is the gimmick—which I believe is basically evil— that keeps the HMO business going."

Is there a difference between doctors who capitate and those who refuse? Apparently yes. A poll taken among 30,000 readers of *Consumer Reports* showed that at Tufts University medical center, which pays most doctors for their services on a fee basis, only four percent of readers complained about not getting sufficient care.

But at three HMOs—Health Net, California Care and Pru Care—who often pay doctors through capitation, up to 19 percent of subscribers said they didn't get the needed care. The same survey showed that 18 percent of readers had to go outside their HMO plan to get the help they believed necessary.

Secret Contracts with Doctors

Patients know nothing of these financial shenanigans, even though they can seriously affect their health care. One reason is that most HMO contracts with doctors stipulate secrecy, including what the doctor is being paid and his financial incentives. Says one WellCare physician's contract: "No materials, pamphlets, or explanatory letters regarding WellCare shall be provided to members." They ask that the doctor refer all such inquiries to the HMOs.

Doctor incentives to ration care are vital to the HMO bottom line. But equally important is the "utilization review" system, which requires that doctors get prior approval from the HMO before embarking on expensive treatment.

Doctors resent this. But so far—until doctors become organized against the HMOs—there's little they can do about this intrusion into their practice of medicine. Ideally, those who authorize treatment would be doctors, or even specialists. But often the authorizers are merely nurses, even clerks, who have been trained to ask nosy questions but don't necessarily understand the answers. And the treatment a patient receives—or doesn't receive—often depends on the whims of these too often undereducated "utilization" people.

Dr. Richard Silver, a noted oncologist at New York Hospital–Cornell Medical School is aghast at the role of interlopers between his medical skill and his patients. A New York daily newspaper printed a portion of his conversation with the "utilization review" person, a nurse working for MetLife's HMO.

She had called Dr. Silver, concerned that the patient, who was suffering from acute leukemia, might be spending too many days in the hospital.

To ensure that people didn't think he had fantasized the forty-five-minute conversation, Dr. Silver taped it. A short excerpt includes the following:

Dr. Silver: "Do you know what the induction regimens for acute leukemia are?"

HMO Nurse: "No, I don't," she admits, adding that her medical director probably does. But, unfortunately, she says, he's not around.

Dr. Silver: "Why isn't he?"

HMO Nurse: "Because I'll explain why, sir. There is a company that is interested in purchasing our insurance plan."

Dr. Silver: "You're trying to sell insurance for profit. I'm trying to save lives."

The Drive for Profits

This draws a crass commercial portrait of managed care, but too often an accurate one. As I've noted, the drive for profits is intense in the HMO world, which now seems more allied with Wall Street than with the medical community.

In fact, HMOs and the stock market are intimately entwined, with no benefit to the patient and probably much to his detriment. The benefits devolve to HMO executives, who will receive higher salaries and extravagant bonuses. And of course it is equally valuable to stockholders in the for-profit HMOs, which includes most of them.

An HMO's quarterly earnings basically determine its stock price, and thus the value of stockholder dividends, if any. If the company is ever sold or merged, both executives and stockholders would receive large capital gains as well.

The compensation to health care executives, who make sixty-two percent *more* than those in other fields, is often scandalous. In one recent year, Leonard Abramson, founder and CEO of U.S. Healthcare, since merged with Aetna, took in $63.2 million in salary, bonuses, and options, only to be outdone by Steve Wiggins, former head of Oxford Health Plans, headquartered in Norwalk, Connecticut, who received $97.2 million.

In free enterprise, one should respect solid CEO compensation, but the greed of health insurance entrepreneurs is still shocking. The year Wiggins received his awesome salary, his remuneration represented fifteen percent of the total premiums paid by subscribers, sick and well!

Even when he failed, Wiggins continued to reap glory payments for his work. Discharged in 1998 when the company had a previous year loss of $291 million, he was given a golden parachute exit. He received a $3.6-million cash payment, plus annual payments of $1.8 million for three years as a "consultant," plus the services of a secretary, dues at the Harvard Club and the Wee Burn Country Club in Darien, Connecticut, along with stock options he can exercise until 2002.

All this on your health insurance premiums.

(At the last moment, the Superintendent of Insurance of New York State ordered a "suspension" of Wiggins's departing package, but it's not clear if officials can interfere in the executive compensation of a stockholder corporation.)

Managed Care is big business, with a gross annual revenue of an estimated $250 billion. Profits in the field vary year to year, but in most years HMOs—including their offshoots, the Preferred Provider Organizations (PPOs) and Point of Service groups (POSs)—took profits of some $20 billion out of the medical care pile.

HMO Execs Get Rich

The pickings of HMO executives are quite rich. Not long ago, one HMO chief, Daniel D. Crowley, head of Foundation Health Corp., voluntarily cut his own mammoth paycheck by $2 million. Before we send consolations, remember that he still took home almost $1.5 million in compensation and reportedly had options worth $10 million.

Graef Crystal, a California pay consultant, points out that the conflict in HMO compensation is philosophical: "There is a problem when these people are slicing care, slicing services, and then making a million dollars."

Senior HMO executives can receive astronomical profits when their firms are bought out or merge, which is increasingly common. In the merger of Health Net and Well Point Health Network, the value of just the Health Net executive's share came to $209 million. Once the merger was completed, the former CEO of Health Systems International, the parent of Health Net, had a personal stake of some $32 million, an awesome sum considering that his original investment was only $300,000, money he put in when he converted the formerly nonprofit HMO into a fully commercial one in 1992.

This is in a field ostensibly dedicated to healing the sick.

Wall Street Favorites

The last decade of HMO growth has been phenomenal, rising from just a handful of subscribers. In 1980 only four percent of the population were enrolled in HMOs. Today, managed health care, in all its many forms, dominates the field of health and health insurance, covering some 130 million Americans.

During this period, the HMO phenomenon has had a profound effect on Wall Street. HMO stocks were the glory boys right up to the mid-1990s, when their stocks moved in only one direction—up. Since then, the general direction of HMO stocks has been down, as earnings either have plummeted or companies have gotten into trouble.

Columbia/HCA, a combined hospital and HMO giant, once a darling of Wall Street, dropped from $45 a share in March 1997 to $26 in October 1997 as the government announced that they were being investigated. Oxford Health Plans, which has grown phenomenally in the number of subscribers, and whose stock had increased from four dollars a share in 1991 to $89 in 1997, suddenly reported enormous losses in late 1997. The stock lost over sixty percent of its value in a single day, shaking the faith of investors who thought the HMO was a perpetual money machine.

More important, these gyrations—reflections of how HMOs price their product and put in restrictions on medical care—affect most of American medicine and dictate how we will be treated when we're sick.

Why? Have the HMOs advanced medical care and provided more efficient ways of delivering it?

Absolutely not. The HMO revolution has been of no value medically; in fact, it has been a distinct detriment. The meager payments by HMOs to university teaching hospitals, for instance, have cut down the schools' ability to do research. In truth, the HMO is not a medical plan at all, but strictly an insurance gimmick.

Only an Insurance Scheme

With the exception of the few which have doctors, clinics, and hospitals of their own, or those sponsored or connected to university hospitals, HMOs are merely insurance schemes that take premiums and redistribute them to providers. They generally do this at a lower rate than private indemnity insurers and keep some twenty percent of the take for themselves for administration, and a sizable profit.

But they operate by exploiting the present network of existing doctors and hospitals, adding nothing to the system.

HMOs claim that they are a positive development because of two factors: the use of preventive medicine and the work of "primary" doctor who supposedly manages all your health care.

These claims are an exaggeration, even a distortion, of reality. The idea that HMOs practice more preventive care than traditional medicine appears to be more spin than reality. That position was easily exploded by *Consumer Reports*, which studied the question and found that HMOs practiced no more preventive medicine than other insurers. In fact, at Oxford, only 13 percent of its diabetic subscribers received a retinal eye exam—a *must* in any preventive care program.

As for the HMO "primary" doctor, he is more rationer and gatekeeper than he is a health manager. He is also quite transient. Americans traditionally like to find one "good doctor" and stay with him. But in the HMO world, many physicians play medical chairs, signing up with one plan, then leaving and joining another. The result is that many HMO "primary" doctors disappear on their patients when they're needed.

One survey showed that fifteen percent of doctors left their HMO plan in the middle of a patient's treatment. In another plan, the turnover rate rose to an incredible thirty percent. That nonhonor went to Humana of South Florida and to Humana Illinois/Indiana.

Even if your own doctor joins the HMO where you are a subscriber, you might not be able to use him, or her, as your primary doctor. This happened to a magazine editor who subscribed to the Oxford plan only to learn that his doctor of eleven years—though an Oxford physician—couldn't see him. Why? The plan prohibited the doctor from taking on any *new* patients.

Then how did the HMOs grow so rapidly? Purely because of low-ball pricing in an era when the national medical budget was rising over ten percent per year, some three times faster than inflation. If we are to place the blame for that—and we should—it rests not only on the expensive new medical technology and the cost of federal programs like Medicare and Medicaid, but on the greed of the medical profession and the pharmaceutical manufacturers, for which we are all now paying heavily.

During the 1970s and 1980s, doctors—fearful of supposedly inevitable socialized medicine—were trying to cash in rapidly before the goose that laid the golden egg choked on its own progeny. Hospitals were expanding so easily that we are now stuck with almost forty percent empty beds, three times more than in Europe. But instead of the bête noire of socialized medicine, the medical profession, and its patients, were faced with an unexpected ogre—the HMO.

The Health Maintenance Organizations—a misnomer if there ever was one—moved quickly into the morass of excessive costs, exploiting the market to the hilt with low premiums to the employer. To businesses, which were involved in steep downsizing and cost cutting themselves, the HMO looked very familiar and was a godsend. The savings became more important than any loss of care or excessive medical controls, things they knew nothing about.

HMOs glossed over, even lied, by not divulging trade secrets, which are now finally coming out. But whatever the shenanigans, the price was seductive to hard-hit businesses that wanted to continue providing some kind of health care for their workers.

The Lure of Lower Premiums

"We have seven employees and a total of ten, including dependents who need medical insurance," says the business manager of a literary agency. "We had excellent private insurance with Blue Cross/Blue Shield and a major medical policy with Phoenix. They didn't question the medical care our people received, and they paid promptly. We had that insurance through 1997, but we were getting regular raises of about ten percent per year. The premiums had finally risen to $55,000 a year and we decided we could no longer afford it. Now, beginning in 1998, we are switching to Oxford. What are we paying? Thirty-three thousand a year—a big difference."

That's how the HMOs became popular. But the low-ball premiums had to be made up for somewhere, and that was in less medical care, restrictions on access, and lower payments to providers.

The initial reaction to HMOs was hosannahs from employers, even from a large number of subscribers who were not sick. But then the counterreaction set in, as some subscribers developed serious and life-threatening illnesses and doctors were hamstrung in treating them—what with both "gatekeepers" and "utilization review" people following the dollar and not the health of patients.

After a while even less than seriously ill patients began to react as their once easy access to specialists was blocked by "gatekeepers" who received bonuses for holding down specialist referrals.

Some patients are unsophisticated and will take any doctor, but the more sophisticated know that once a primary doctor screens you and suspects an illness, whether diabetes, a cardiac condition, hypertension, or cancer, a board-certified specialist is the *only* physician qualified to treat you. The nuances of modern medicine are not sufficiently known to family doctors, nor is the enormous panoply of medications for each illness, including their benefits and side effects.

The HMO "gatekeeper" is no longer considered the physician who should manage your total care and provide information and planning. Instead he is increasingly seen in his true light—as the person who would, consciously or otherwise, limit your access to superior care and procedures in order to save money for the HMO.

HMO "Freedom" Plans

Dissatisfaction with traditional HMOs created the relatively new and increasingly popular "freedom" or full-access HMO plans. They cost more, but they allow the patient to see specialists without prior approval.

This does not eliminate the other HMO drawbacks—the evils of bonuses for reduced care, the intrusion of the "utilization review" for prior approval of treatments, or the shifting of responsibility within the "capitation" business. But it does give the patient more freedom to move around in the complex medical world, generally the best way for patients to find the proper doctor, treatment, and hospital in situations of serious illness.

"We've taken the Oxford Freedom Plan so that our employees can better manage their own care," says the literary agency business manager. "It increases our premiums, and our people have to pay more out-of-pocket. First there's a five-hundred-dollar deductible each year per employee, and then there's a twenty percent co-payment on medical bills. But for us it's worth the extra money. It's still much cheaper than the private insurance we had before."

These "freedom" plans, which are generally called POSs—Point of Service in the industry—but are still HMOs to the public, are the most popular new innovations. But we have yet to see how they will truly fare, whether the HMO horror stories will continue, and whether the employers can afford them any more than they did the fee-for-service indemnity plans.

We also have yet to see whether the HMOs can afford them. Perhaps not, which would sink the entire movement. Oxford Health Plans, as mentioned, recently woke up to find out that it was $200 million in arrears in payments to doctors and hospitals, much of it created by their new freedom system. Recently, Oxford took over a billion-dollar loss to make up for its failed projections of its costs, especially for its popular "freedom" plan.

The Rising Costs of HMOs

As patients are somewhat able to circumvent their "gate-keepers," and the onetime gain from HMO price "low-balling" becomes history, the costs of the HMOs are rising, and their prices are rising as well. Kaiser, for one, has announced a quarter of a billion loss for 1997, a sign that the low premiums that gained HMOs such easy acceptance among employers were faulty.

Now, HMO premiums are beginning to rise again. In 1998 several HMOs have already asked for anywhere from five to ten percent hikes in their rates to meet rising costs. In addition, doctors may start to rebel against the HMOs and organize, both to increase their fees and to get paid more rapidly than the industry average of two months plus.

The overall result is that medical costs nationally are going up. For three years, from 1994 through 1996, costs were rising less than inflation, but those days are over. Costs in 1998 seem to have gone up almost five percent, with dire warnings for 1999 and beyond that we might again see double-digit medical inflation.

The Center for Survey Research estimates that 1999 health inflation will come in between 4.5 and 8 percent, much higher than regular inflation. At the upper range, that eliminates much of the temporary gains from the HMO "revolution."

"It's pent-up cost pressure," says Stephen Karp of Ryder Systems, Inc. "Insurers will take a deep breath and pass on some of their increased costs to consumers."

Other casualties of the once-again rising medical costs

are the poor, and even the aged. The major HMOs, including Aetna, U.S. Healthcare, and several Blue Cross and Blue Shield plans, have shut down service to Medicaid patients in twelve states—including New York, New Jersey, Connecticut, Florida, Massachusetts, and California. In Ohio and California, HMOs are curtailing services in some countries to Medicare patients as well.

Doctors Lose As Well

One casualty of the HMO revolution has been doctor incomes, which although still rising are no longer going up the way they once did. Although new figures published in 1998 indicate they are becoming star earners again, there's a great deal of bitterness, especially among specialists and surgical subspecialists who gave much of the élan to sophisticated modern medicine (see Chapter VI).

"Since the dominance of the HMOs, my income has fallen forty percent," says a bitter orthopedic surgeon in Stamford, Connecticut. "They pay me at least a third less than the private insurers did, and they try to tell you how to practice medicine. I'm lucky that I'm ending my medical career soon and not starting it. I wouldn't have tolerated the HMOs. But today, I have no choice. Without them, I couldn't make a good living practicing medicine."

Specialists are especially angered at the HMO revolution, which, in a way, has pitted them against primary doctors, on whom they must rely for referrals in most HMO plans. One otolaryngologist in New York complains that the HMO "gatekeepers" are keeping him from practicing quality medicine. He tells the story of a neighbor who rushed into his office with her daughter. The child had fallen on a shard of glass and was bleeding profusely:

"After I stopped the bleeding and sutured the laceration, my neighbor produced her insurance card—for an HMO. She called the pediatrician's office to request a referral, but he refused, claiming she should have brought the child to him. My office assistant also failed to obtain the referral. The patient returned to have the stitches removed, and I obliged—although the pediatrician again refused to make a referral. Neither bill was ever paid."

The HMO's Idealistic Beginnings

To give credit where it belongs, the health maintenance field started out altruistically enough. It was not so much to make big money, but to provide better care in a "managed" setting. Its birthplace was in the so-called "group practices," which were supposed to join physicians together, both geographically and spiritually, and do five things:

1. Take care of the whole patient by having both primary and specialty doctors on the same premises, creating a "group." They would be attached to a quality hospital, or ideally have one of their own.
2. Do full preventive maintenance with regular exams, immunizations, education, etc.
3. Provide patients with the most modern care, as doctors would be sharing knowledge, both of the patient and of medicine in general.
4. Establish each patient with his own primary doctor, who would supervise all his care.
5. Reduce the cost of medicine through shared facilities and equipment.

The model launched such entities as the Health Insurance Plan of New York (HIP, which still exists), created to care for city employees in the 1930s. That was followed by the Kaiser Permanente plan, started to provide health care for workers building a dam in the California desert, then expanded to Kaiser shipyard workers during World War II.

These plans, especially Kaiser, closely followed the original group idea. Kaiser put its doctors on salary so there would be no economic incentives for excess care, and even built clinics and hospitals in California. Though they priced their care somewhat below that of indemnity insurance companies to attract subscribers, their medical work was considered excellent.

Most of today's HMOs, including some of Kaiser's, have little to do with the original concept of group medicine. The ideal was soon distorted, giving birth only to cheaper insurance rather than better medicine.

Are All HMOs Medical Rackets?

Should we paint all HMOs with the same brush? Are there any good ones? Naturally, in any field there are stars, institutions for whom the excellence of medicine is more important than the bottom line. Almost invariably these are nonprofit HMOs, including many that started out idealistically. They include Health Partners in Minneapolis, Harvard Pilgrim Health Plan in Boston, and Group Health of Puget Sound, among others, all developed around the original "group" ideal.

To this day, the nonprofits still provide better service overall, spending a larger share of the premium dollar on medical care.

(Many of these, however, are yielding to bigness. Both Health Partners and Puget Sound have just been swallowed up by the giant of nonprofits, the Kaiser system.)

The whole theory of contemporary HMOs is flawed, but the public has invested in it heavily and is concerned about which ones are better. Generally, if not always, the nonprofits come out on top. *Modern Maturity* magazine, for instance, in comparing HMOs, tells two anecdotes, one of inferior and one of superior care.

In California's Lucerne Valley, a retired person explains that he suffers from high blood pressure and cataracts. He had a pituitary tumor removed from his brain in 1990, when he was covered by an indemnity policy from his former employer. In 1993 he retired and joined an HMO because it was cheaper.

From then on it was a continual fight. First, his HMO

didn't want to give him the regular hormones he required because of the pituitary operation. Worse yet, they refused to cover the periodic MRI screenings required to check if his tumor had grown back.

"Their little trick," says the disgruntled patient, "is that they just don't answer. If you ask to see a specialist, they just don't answer you, or if you need a test, they don't answer you."

Disgusted, he finally quit the HMO and went back to his old, more expensive indemnity policy. He got his MRI screening, only to learn that the tumor had grown back. He is now on radiation treatment.

This is exactly the opposite story of a retired elevator operator who for fifteen years has been enrolled in Boston's nonprofit Harvard Pilgrim Health Plan. A former smoker, he has suffered from emphysema for twenty-five years, and four years ago had lung cancer surgery, including an operation to reduce the size of his diseased lungs. Most of the work was done at a first-rate university teaching hospital in Boston, where he has also had cataract surgery and now faces another operation to remove a growth from his throat.

Although he has had a few tiffs with the plan, he credits them with his survival. This retiree had the benefit of an older, more idealistic nonprofit HMO connected with a university hospital. Not too many HMO subscribers can tell the same story.

HMOs Are a Washington Creation

Surprisingly, the HMO revolution was launched by the federal government itself in the 1970s, in order to invite the private sector to take over medical care instead of Washington. The intellectual impetus came from the Jackson Hole study group, headed by a former pediatric neurologist, Dr. Paul Elwood, Jr., who had been a hospital director.

At the time, Dr. Elwood—who recently lamented that

the HMO revolution has been taken out of the hands of doctors—was angry that indemnity insurance policies, which dominated the field, were paying doctors and hospitals very generously but were pinching pennies on preventive care. He organized a series of conferences at his home in Jackson Hole, Wyoming, which were attended by politicians, physicians, and assorted policy gurus interested in medical reform. It was Dr. Elwood who coined the phrase "Health Maintenance Organization," or HMO, a play on the concept of preventive, or whole, medicine.

His work came to the attention of President Nixon, who saw in the HMO the chance of a medical revolution that relied on the private sector and not on the government, which some feared might someday promote socialized medicine. The cost savings of Elwood's utopian concept of prepaid groups also appealed to the White House, and to the corporate people who attended his confabs.

In 1973 the Department of Health, Education and Welfare reprinted a forty-year-old document drafted by the Committee on the Costs of Medical Care. The appeal of preventive medicine and lower costs promoted in that report was irresistible, and even though HMOs at the time served only two percent of the population, Congress gave its official imprimatur.

In December of that year, Congress passed the Health Maintenance Act of 1973, which not only allotted $375 million to get HMOs launched, but preempted state laws that prohibited medical groups that took in prepaid premiums from subscribers. It went further: it required companies of twenty-five or more employees to offer a "federally qualified HMO plan" to their workers.

False Claims of Efficiency

One claim of HMO theorists was not only that they would cut costs, but would be more *efficient*. In reality, the HMO system as it has developed is the least efficient, most fragmented, of all medical care entities. Instead, HMOs have created a mammoth bureaucracy with various parts of medical care scattered by geography, and with approvals required all along the way. It is the opposite, for instance, of the more efficient university hospital system, where staff faculty doctors and residents, and various departments, coordinate the patient's care.

A pediatrician from the Los Angeles area, Dr. Gary F. Krieger, wrote of his frustrations with HMOs: "Efficiency, in my opinion has clearly decreased, not increased. Every day I hear complaints from my colleagues and from my patients about the increased time involved in treatment. . . . I'm familiar with the controls of HMOs. I have yet to experience the benefits."

He tells of a seriously ill diabetic child he wanted to hospitalize. He ordered a lab workup, only to learn that the HMO involved required that the family drive twenty miles to a lab they had under contract—even though there were plenty of local labs. He called in an endocrinologist, who, once he saw the lab report, wanted to admit the child to the hospital, but learned that he didn't have the power. The HMO had approved the specialist, but only for a consultation.

Dr. Krieger finally got permission for hospitalization, but the HMO computer broke down, adding hours of delay. In all, he says, "what would have taken me only one to two hours in previous days took me almost twenty-four hours to accomplish. That is not what I call efficient."

In another case of his, that of a fourteen-month-old baby with a cleft palate and lip, Dr. Krieger had to conquer a medical HMO maze before the child could be helped. The parents came to his office, proud that the father had gotten a good job. He was off Medicaid and was now covered by an HMO. The baby was scheduled to undergo a third operation at the county hospital to complete the repair of the cleft palate. But now that the family was no longer on Medicaid, the county hospital needed approval from the HMO.

The HMO refused. They stated that it had no contract with the county hospital. Instead, their physicians would reevaluate the child and see if further repair of her condition was called for.

The distraught father quit his job and got back on Medicaid so his child could get the operation. In all, the process took six months, not five days.

"The system [HMO] is fundamentally flawed," says Dr. Krieger, who excepts only those who have physicians on salary in a hospital-doctor complex. "However, for the majority of physicians practicing in this country, managed care is placing impediments in getting service for patients."

Another negative aspect of HMOs is their *excessive* drive to limit the time patients spend in hospitals. In the HMO world, actuarial firms, not individual doctors, increasingly make these decisions. One prominent firm that consults for several HMOs is Milliman & Robertson of Seattle, who work for CIGNA and Kaiser Permanente. They have compiled eight volumes of guidelines to advise doctors how long patients should stay in the hospital.

Bone infections in children? Two days can be enough. Mastectomies for women with breast cancer? It can even be done outpatient. M & R is the firm that once pronounced that cataract surgery on one eye was enough—that you needn't see well out of two eyes! Dr. Robert Yetman, their pediatric consultant, even suggested that children with heart valve infections be sent home after three days, which raised the medical ire. "When you send a child home, who's going to manage treatment?" asks Dr. Thomas Cleary, infectious disease expert at the University of Texas.

HMOs Seek Out Medicare Patients

Cutting down costs is the first priority, but the latest movement—or impediment—in the HMO field is the recruiting of Medicare patients. Some seniors are switching to HMOs because of financial inducements: they need not put up the $100 deductible each year, nor the $760 deductible when they are hospitalized, or the twenty percent co-payment for doctors. Some HMOs include part or full prescription coverage, and even eyeglasses. Some HMOs advertise that seniors can even drop their Medigap insurance.

Some seniors do switch to save money. At present that represents one in six Medicare patients, with the percentage rising. However, in certain states, including California, Arizona, Oregon, and others, the percentage of seniors enrolled in HMOs is much higher. Observers believe those who sign up are generally healthy and don't worry about giving up the unlimited fee-for-service care provided by regular Medicare.

The HMOs have been accused of "cherry-picking" the healthy seniors and avoiding the sick ones. One way they accomplish this is through "Medicare Breakfast" solicitations, to which seniors are invited to hear why they should drop their present unlimited coverage and accept the restrictive HMO plan. The trick here is that by inviting only the obviously ambulatory aged to the free breakfast, they eliminate the house-bound or hospitalized seniors. Also, HMO plans know that generally it is the healthiest senior who would risk losing his normal coverage.

It is truly a financial bonanza for HMOs. The federal government pays them ninety-five percent of what the typical senior coverage would cost—an average of some $6,000—all the way up to $9,000 a year. But the "cherry-picked" enrollees cost the plans much less, granting them huge profits.

HMOs Are Risky for Medicare Patients

The seniors who do sign up, critics say, are taking a grave risk with their insurance. These seniors, particularly healthy sixty-five-year-olds, forget that as they approach seventy-five and eighty, most will develop serious ailments, some of which will require constant care. Under conventional Medicare, they are fully protected and have the freedom to manage their own case—to locate the best doctors and treatment available, including so-called "experimental" therapies at top hospitals. That's a privilege, perhaps the best medical system in the nation, that they should not easily give up.

Right now the government is trying to push seniors into HMOs in order to eventually save money. But switching to a Medicare HMO could be an unwise insurance risk for the patient. The government now permits seniors to switch back and forth from traditional coverage to HMOs, but that could change as Washington starts to run out of Medicare funds.

About one-fifth of the seniors who switch to HMOs eventually leave, but that number could rise as more discover their mistake. The General Accounting Office tells of a case of an elderly HMO enrollee who had ankle surgery. Fourteen days after his discharge from the hospital, he was diagnosed as suffering from a lack of oxygen in his blood. "The elderly enrollee was not readmitted to the hospital until two days after the diagnosis was made, and died on the day of admission."

Several HMO Medicare patients are suing the government for failing to take action when their HMO—Family Health Plan—allegedly denied them needed treatment. According to her lawyers, the patients had the following complaints:

- A seventy-one-year-old woman with diabetes, high blood pressure and congestive heart failure, had her right leg amputated at the knee after her HMO doctors failed to respond to complaints of pain in her foot.
- When a woman broke her hip at home, the HMO allegedly refused to pay for an ambulance, and her daughter had to drive the injured woman to the hospital. Though the emergency room X rays allegedly showed possible multiple fractures, she was refused admission to the hospital.
- A woman in a nursing home who was being treated for pneumonia was allegedly discharged by

her doctor. Says the complaint: "At this point, the patient was receiving medication for pneumonia and was in such great pain that she could not walk, eat, or use the toilet."

New Medicare Regulations

Because of the federal/private drive to enroll more seniors in HMOs, Medicare, beginning in August 1998, put in some new regulations to protect against excessive HMO exploitation:

- Women may demand direct access to gynecologists for routine and preventive care.
- All patients with *severe* or *chronic* ailments must be allowed direct access to specialists in *some* cases, e.g., chemotherapy for cancer.
- Patients can demand information on how the HMO pays its doctors.
- Emergency room care must be provided when a *prudent* person thinks it is necessary.
- If care is denied by an HMO, the patient has the right to swift appeal to an independent board of experts.
- If a patient believes he should stay in the hospital, he will be able to, without charge, while his complaint about being evicted is arbitrated.

It all sounds good, but it still falls far short of the present non-HMO Medicare plan, which—with a Medigap policy—is among the best health insurance in the nation.

The government is being unconscionable in encouraging seniors to join HMOs in order to save a few pennies while it squanders trillions in other areas.

Doctors Also Taking a Risk with HMOs

Doctors who "capitate" their Medicare HMO patients in order to increase their income are also taking a risk. In their case, it is an insurance one. They receive considerably more from Medicare than for other patients. It can be a windfall for doctors hard-pressed to make their conventional bundle of $250,000 to $350,000 a year on regular HMO and Medicare fees. But, experts warn, if a physician handles too many Medicare seniors for an HMO, and has to pay for several major illnesses out of the capitation money, his financial well could run dry.

Internist Allen Smith, medical director of a nine-physician group in Massachusetts, warns that doctors should be careful how many seniors they take on: "If too much of your income is dependent on Medicare HMOs, and you're not good at managing care, you could be over your head very quickly."

Another caveat—more important to patients—is that some doctors might skimp on services to seriously ill Medicare HMO patients when pressed, in order to make ends meet.

HMOs Crack Down Further

Recently, large HMOs, including Aetna U.S. Healthcare, which has almost 14 million subscribers, have further reduced fees paid to doctors in order to increase the bottom line. Physicians are balking and complaining to state insurance commissions, but usually fruitlessly. A review of 100 HMO-doctor contracts reviewed by the AMA showed that, increasingly, HMOs can lower fees at will without consulting the doctor. For the patient this means less time and attention from their physicians.

Along with Aetna, Blue Cross and Blue Shield plans are also cutting fees. One New York ophthalmologist said Aetna had cut his follow-up exams to $27 from $70. Doctors can complain, but in most contracts they have given up their right to sue the HMO.

Patients are in an even worse bind. The original federal law that helped set up the HMOs in the 1970s (ERISA) protected managed care plans from lawsuits from patient-subscribers. If care is denied to a patient by the insurer, the patient can sue the doctor for malpractice but cannot sue the HMO. (One court decision in Texas held up patients' rights to sue HMOs, but that is an isolated case.)

Some doctors are so frustrated with HMOs that they drop out and try to set up their own managed care plans—usually unsuccessfully. In a noble experiment to beat the HMOs, the California Medical Association and 7,500 of its member-physicians decided to take on that state's giant HMOs. Called California Advantage, it set as its goal "putting patients first and profits second." "They had a very well intentioned and very naïve strategy," says an Oakland health consultant, pointing out that they went up against financial behemoths with only a few million dollars. In 1998, California Advantage went bankrupt.

One such plan, in Connecticut, did succeed, but greed eventually did that in. "M.D. Health Plan" was established in 1986 by the Connecticut State Medical Society and 3,000 physicians. It became the state's second largest plan, with 161,000 subscribers, but in 1995, the doctors sold out to an HMO for $101 million—15 times their original investment.

The New York State Medical Society refuses to enter the fray, but Kansas, Louisiana, and Pennsylvania, where HMO competition is reportedly weaker, are going to try to wrest control back into medical hands. Nationwide, the chances are slim for doctor-managed medicine *unless* laws are changed to weaken HMOs' often abusive power.

Individual Insurees

In the HMO world (as with some other insurers), the truly odd man out is still the individual, the person who belongs to no group and may be self-employed. For the longest time they have been discriminated against by having to pay exorbitant premiums that are constantly being raised. Oxford, for one, recently requested a giant increase for individual insurees. One Manhattan real estate agent was notified that her premiums would rise from $324 a month to $547, a massive 69 percent increase.

This category of "individual insuree" is quite large and includes those who have lost their jobs and their coverage, or have switched jobs, plus some who are sick and unwanted by insurers who "cherry-pick" their subscribers in order to eliminate the higher risks. Some of the most vulnerable are those with preexisting medical conditions, from diabetes to cancer to heart disease.

Since no insurer wants them, Congress and the president united with great hoopla to supposedly solve this problem. The Kassebaum-Kennedy bill passed in 1996 was designed to grant health insurance to everyone who wanted it, sick or not, employed or not. By mandating that insurance companies cover these outcasts, it was believed that salvation for these uninsured was now at hand.

The only problem was that the federal government didn't mention price. In March 1998, after a survey of the field, the General Accounting Office announced, in effect, that the legislation was a near fiasco. The newly eligible couldn't afford to pay the price put on this insurance. Premiums for those individuals ranged up to 600 percent higher than those for standard policies! In some cases, the cost was $15,000 a year and more.

Despite Uncle Sam's hulabaloo, the industry is frank about the fact that they still don't want the individual insuree. American Medical Security, one insurer, said they reserve the right to charge these "high-risk" individuals *five times the normal rate.* Some federal bill. Some insurance.

Finally, in response to the outcry, the White House has announced that it will penalize any HMO that doesn't insure sick individuals by removing their right to insure federal employees.

In New York State, in response to HMO price increases for individual insurees, Governor Pataki announced that the state would pick up the tab by paying the insurance companies *over $100 million* so that they wouldn't have to raise those rates.

The action is generous but ridiculous. In true insurance logic, the risk of the sick should be spread out over the entire geographic population of the area. That way everyone is insured at *reasonable*, not exorbitant, rates. But in the stockholder-owned for-profit HMOs, the only logic is quarterly bottom lines and their Wall Street stock price—poor critera for better health.

How Good Is Your HMO?

How good is your HMO, or the one you might soon be pushed into, either by your employer or the government?

The industry is trying to set up at least minimum standards through an organization called the National Committee for Quality Assurance (NCQA), ostensibly a totally independent accrediting group for HMOs. So far, less than half the 651 HMOs (they don't count PPOs or POSs) are accredited or being investigated. But the figures are not very reassuring as to quality.

Only 157 are fully accredited for three years; ninety-one for one year; ten have only "provisional" one-year accreditation; and twelve have been denied. Some are not accredited because they don't care enough to apply or are afraid that they would be denied. They rely on advertising and price to attract their employer-clients, and for most employees it's take what you get—or else. Of course, subscribers should find out if their HMO is accredited, and if not, try to switch to a better plan, if that exists.

You can learn if your HMO plan is accredited by calling 1-888-275-7585.

Or you can find the full list, including the "denied"

plans, on the Internet website at www.ncqa.org. If you're low-tech, you can write for the list to the National Committee for Quality Assurance at 2000 L Street, NW, Washington, D.C. 20036, and enclose ten dollars.

The NCQA has developed a quality gauge called HEDIS (Health Employer Data and Information Set), which ostensibly measures quality performance in the hope this standard will be adopted nationwide, like the accreditation program for hospitals. And the hope is that employers, and patients, will begin to trust it.

But some people, unsure if the NCQA organization is impartial, are skeptical. Some even hint that the HEDIS measurement was developed to protect the HMO industry. That's the opinion of Catherine Kunkle, vice-president of the National Business Coalition on Health, who also serves on the HEDIS review committee.

"There's a lot of resistance to expanding that report card," she says, "and the danger is that HEDIS may produce a report card that is so minimal that it just won't have much credibility."

Solutions to the HMO Crisis

Meanwhile, without any assurances of quality care, and with considerable suspicion in the opposite direction, the HMO industry is still growing rapidly:

. . . despite the rising costs and competition that have hit the bottom line of many HMOs in 1997 and devastated their stock prices. (In fact, half the HMOs lost money in 1997.) As a result, they are being forced to reevaluate their system and what they have to charge employers to stay in business.

. . . despite the fact that "freedom" plans have emboldened HMO subscribers to rebel against having to use a network of doctors and no one else. Perhaps most irritating to patients is the need for their "gatekeeper" to approve a visit to a specialist.

. . . despite physicians carping about HMOs influencing their practice of medicine and about the *discount* fees they are receiving. Increasingly, there is talk of doctors organizing against the HMOs, a movement that might be led by local medical societies. The AMA is presently just grumbling, but we can expect more concrete action in the near future if doctors are not paid more, if not as much as they made in the heyday of open fee-for-service.

Meanwhile, the present crisis—or more likely, the chaos—of medicine has not been aided by the growth of the HMO movement, except to show that so-called "health maintenance organizations" in their present form are not the answer to quality care delivered at a reasonable price.

As in the case of new federal regulations aimed at greater freedom for Medicare patients enrolled in HMOs, Congress is preparing a "Patient's Bill of Rights" to partially correct the abuses of HMOs.

This could be a step forward in shaping better medical care, but it is very far from the ultimate answer.

What is that answer? For that the reader must be patient, and await "A Plan for Tomorrow" (See Chapter VIII).

Meanwhile, we must tolerate the HMOs in some form for they have filled a market niche created by costs that were rising too rapidly. We cannot totally reform the HMOs, for the theory behind them is flawed. But until the time when the nation becomes sophisticated enough to develop an insurance system that is not tied to either Wall Street or Washington, we suggest the following twelve-point program to reform the HMOs. These must be put into effect by *law* to be of value.

I. All subscribers must have immediate access to specialists without the intervention of the "gatekeeper."

II. There should be no "capitation" payments to doctors, many of whom are tempted to hold back services so they can keep a lion's share of the prepaid money.

III. HMOs should not be permitted to hold back ("withhold") any portion of a doctor's fee, and thus force him to offer less services to his patients in order to retrieve the remainder of his money.

IV. In case of emergencies, patients in the HMO system should be fully covered at *any* emergency room in the nation, rather than only those with whom their HMO has a contract. This rule should also apply, without any challenge, to subscribers who are away from home.

V. HMOs must provide complex care for the seriously ill without claiming that a remedy is "experimental." Standard treatment should be any remedy that is routinely used in university hospitals and in such specialized institutions as the Memorial Sloan-Kettering Cancer Center.

VI. HMOs should be declared a public utility by state governments and governed with as much force as telephone, cable, electric, and gas businesses.

VII. Rather than appeal to the HMO if any medical care is denied, patients shall have immediate recourse to an independent ombudsman organization set up for their protection by each state government.

VIII. Accreditation by an independent medical group shall be necessary for any HMO to operate anywhere in the United States. This group should, by law, not be connected or supported by the HMO industry. The accreditation list should be openly published and sent to all employers and subscribers.

IX. No HMO shall be permitted to have a closed "network" of doctors to whom the patient *must go*, unless that HMO has a central medical center, including an accredited hospital and doctors on salary, such as the

Mayo Clinic, the Cleveland Clinic, or a university teaching medical center staffed by the faculty.

X. A state board of review to control HMOs shall be headed by a person elected by the people of the state. The present overview by an insurance commissioner is not sufficient protection for subscribers in a system where *less* medical care is the equation that makes for *more* HMO profits.

XI. "Gag rules" shall be illegal, and no contract between a doctor and an HMO shall include any oath of loyalty or pledge of secrecy, except to the patient.

XII. The state of Minnesota now prohibits "for-profit" HMOs from operating in that state. Its eleven HMOs are all nonprofit groups such as Blue Cross/Blue Shield. Other states should take similar legal action.

The current HMO mess was created by excessive costs stimulated, as I have said, by the greed of doctors, hospitals, pharmaceutical companies, and other suppliers. Into that void came the even greater greed of HMOs and their exploitation of medical services for giant profits.

The situation can only be remedied by reforming the HMOs, then by implementing a better system of health insurance in the United States, one which we will discuss in the conclusion of this book. The public expects, and deserves, quality medical choice at a reasonable price—not what they're now receiving from the flawed HMOs.

Chapter II

The American Hospital

Center of Healing or Horror?

The forty-six-year-old mother of two had just undergone a hysterectomy in a Cincinnati hospital and was struggling with severe pain. Surprisingly, it was not in her lower abdomen at the site of her incision, but in the upper portion. The woman complained again and again and the "nurse" wrote down that it was "incisional pain," which was incorrect.

After three days of this, as her blood pressure dropped and her temperature rose dangerously, doctors who were now involved suspected the worst. During surgery, her bowel had been nicked and leaking feces had created a massive infection. She died two days later.

Eventually, the hospital settled the lawsuit for $3 million, but the verdict had a special significance. The patient had not been attended by a registered nurse, but by a "patient care technician," one of the many euphemisms now given by hospitals to laypeople with only weeks of training who can be expected to make such mistakes. A registered nurse probably would have noticed the difference early on and alerted the doctor. Just the simple difference of life or death.

The American hospital is regaled with praise, even glorified on television as millions watch miracles unfold before their eyes. Some of that is quite true, as modern technology and dedicated staffs save lives almost on schedule.

The Dark Side of Hospital Care

But like the woman with the deadly infection, those same hospitals are threatened by a multitude of problems that are much less explored and for which—as of now—there seem to be few answers in progress. The situation is worsened because too many hospitals rest on their laurels, seemingly oblivious to the darker side of their care and the mayhem it causes each day.

Everyone hears of the individual horror stories played up by the press—of doctors amputating the wrong limb, cutting the wrong side of someone's brain, taking out the healthy instead of the diseased lung. This is all quite true. But the *real* problem is much deeper, that of a systematic set of errors, negligence, and mistakes that threaten many more lives than the layman can possibly imagine.

The dark side of hospital care is known to *some* members of the medical profession, but even in that sophisticated environment there is a great deal of ignorance about the truth—of the daily threats to good medicine in our 6,200 hospitals. A study of the studies by the finest investigators in the field confirm that these threats are legion.

- Infections are rife, killing many more patients than most people believe. Patients are threatened by a variety of germs, especially the antibiotic-resistant "staph" (staphylococcus), which stubbornly inhabits the wards and surgical suites, causing disease and death.

- To save money, "aides" with various titles but without much training are taking the place of registered nurses with extensive training.
- Medication errors and reactions are much too common, with a much higher level of danger than anyone had believed.
- The quality of care varies enormously from hospital to hospital nationwide, with no overall professional attempt to make it more uniform.
- Mistakes reported in more recent surveys indicate that far more are made in hospitals than it had been assumed; these errors are a leading cause of death.
- The nation has a surplus of hospitals, resulting in an excessive number of empty beds, causing grave financial strain.
- As competition increases and HMO payments decrease, many voluntary or community hospitals are forced to sell to "proprietary" or "for-profit" institutions, or to combine with other institutions.
- Much surgery, as we shall later see, is still unnecessary and medically uncalled for.

Iatrogenic Disease

One of the tragic facts about the modern hospital is that one of the gravest dangers to the patient comes from an unexpected source—the hospital itself, its doctors and nurses. The result is what is called "iatrogenic" disease, the word *iatros* being the Greek term for physician. Whether as a result of infections, drugs, or medical error, the hospital setting endangers a major principle of medicine—*Primum Non Nocere*—"First Do No Harm."

Some harm is inevitable in the modern medical system of aggressive intervention, which overall creates more benefit than damage. But studies indicate that the typical hospital patient is threatened with considerably more damage than he expects.

To take the least conservative view, the patient takes a sizable and often unnecessary gamble every time he enters a hospital. If America's hospitals, including some of our most highly touted ones, would apply greater safeguards of care, what some categorize as an "epidemic" of iatrogenic disease might be eliminated.

The first hospital studies in this field were highly discouraging. In 1964, at Yale–New Haven Hospital, the medical arm of the Yale University School of Medicine, chief resident Dr. Elihu M. Schimmel decided to inventory the negative effects of medical treatment. He studied all the patients who came through what was then the eighty-bed, three-ward Yale Medical Service. After eight months he and his colleagues tallied the results.

The study shook the foundations of the profession. He learned that "noxious responses to medical care" were much higher than physicians, or patients, had expected. Of the 1,014 patients, there were "240 iatrogenic episodes" occurring in 198 patients—a twenty percent failure of good care. According to his report in the *Annals of Internal Medicine*, not only were one in five patients made ill by medical treatment, but it caused or contributed to more than one in ten of all hospital deaths!

"During the course of the study, 154 of the 1,014 patients admitted to the medical service died in the hospital," Schimmel states. "Of these, sixteen deaths were related to noxious episodes. . . ."

The "episodes" struck patients from every direction. Among the 240 there were 31 reactions to blood transfusions; 29 accidents in biopsy and endoscopy (examination of the body's interior with an instrument); 23 infections acquired in the hospital, resulting in 5 deaths; 119 drug reactions; 24 untoward reactions to therapeutic techniques; and 14 miscellaneous hazards.

In an important way, the study underestimated the damage because it *did not count any known errors* made by doctors and nurses or any complications following surgery and anesthesia.

Despite that, if Schimmel's figures are correct—and they come from his firsthand on-the-spot study—then the national mayhem of iatrogenic disease is frightening. It shows that ten percent of the deaths were hospital-created, and that 1.5 percent of all admitted patients died because of medical intervention.

Massive Number of "Noxious Episodes" Nationally

That translates into massive numbers nationwide. Since there were 35 million hospital admissions that year, some 500,000 people may have died in the hospital as a result of unwise drug and medical intervention. These numbers may be even larger, considering that Yale–New Haven Hospital is a superior institution. Not a very safe environment.

The startling study, reported thirty years ago in my book *The Doctors*, was confirmed by similar work at Johns Hopkins, with similar results. Dr. Leighton Cluff, along with the U.S. Public Health Service, studied 718 patients in the Johns Hopkins Osler Service over a three-month period and confirmed the harm and death caused by one element—prescription drugs—in the Yale study.

But, critics point out, the Yale study was done a long time ago, some thirty-five years. Surely the profession has learned and cleaned up its act. It has become more quality-control-oriented, especially in its major hospitals. Hasn't it?

Apparently not. In 1981, Dr. K. Steel came to the same negative conclusion about the state of our hospitals after observing 815 patients in a university teaching institution. Reporting in the *New England Journal of Medicine*, he concluded that more than one-third—thirty-six percent—had an iatrogenic illness caused by treatment, and that almost one in ten patients had an unwanted iatrogenic episode that was either life-threatening or had produced a disability!

The public and the profession were aghast, worrying about the safety and efficiency of our hospitals. But as time went on, they relaxed, assuring themselves that tighter controls were righting the situation. Reportedly, peer review groups in hospitals were clamping down on sloppy procedures. The result, they said, was that hospitals, physicians, and nurses were greatly improving their performance.

The Supposedly "Good News"

Less than ten years ago, from Harvard, came "good news," apparently solid confirmation that America's hospitals were indeed shaping up, and that patients had little to be concerned about. The doors of America's hospitals were not only entry points for the most modern treatments, the public was assured, but the inside of the institutions were safe for patients.

Confirmation of that upbeat view ostensibly came in 1990 from the Harvard Medical Practice Study. It concentrated on 30,121 patients from a number of hospitals in New York, surely a large enough sample to be accurate. But this study was not done on the spot, as were the others. Instead, the Harvard group used only medical records, as if what was officially written down by physicians represented what was truly going on.

That, as we were to learn, is a naive, almost childish attitude to anyone truly familiar with the problems of the medical establishment.

The supposedly upbeat result? There was 3.7 percent adverse reactions to treatment, only a fifth the harm shown by other studies. To be considered "adverse," two physicians had to agree.

The profession now felt better. Yes, America's hospitals were not only modern, but safe.

Of course, there were also skeptics. The Harvard study

was secondhand, coming from records, as we've pointed out, and not from on-the-spot checks. Perhaps the truth would come out if *nonphysicians* were involved in doing the observing, listening to doctors and checking each case in real time. For then there would be little opportunity to conceal the truth—for doctors to *pretend* that all was well.

That's exactly what happened in Chicago not long ago.

The Actual News Is Very Bad

The medical director of a large teaching hospital found himself as a patient in his own institution, a practice that provides insight often unattainable in any other way. All the talk of his hospital being "safe" flew out of his consciousness when he started to experience, firsthand, the lot of patients.

One event especially shook his confidence. He suffered from a food allergy, yet was offered the offending food at his bedside. He turned it away, only to have it come back again, and again. Three times he sent the food back, explaining that it could be dangerous for him.

Now a skeptic, the director called in a professor at the nearby Chicago-Kent College of Law and proposed opening his institutions to them in a unique way. He wanted a survey of iatrogenic in-house harm that was to be conducted on the spot and not from medical records.

Headed by Professor Lori B. Andrews, this study of the unnamed major hospital attached to a Chicago university medical school covered all the patients in ten surgical services. The team of four observers, trained ethnographers, were given unprecedented access to the minute-by-minute operation of the hospital.

They were ever-present on the wards, right alongside as doctors, residents, and interns made their rounds. The observers attended case conferences and any meetings that involved patient care, including meetings on morbidity and mortality, quality of care, even changes of nursing shifts. For nine months they were underfoot, always listening and watching. They recorded the evidence and comments on adverse reactions, then put it all together into a report.

"Observers did not ask questions, and they did not make medical judgments," the report states. "They recorded what was said by health care professionals about the event in that setting." In effect, it was the physicians—through the observers—who were filling in the true facts.

It was all published in *Lancet*, the leading British medical journal, in February 1997. The study came to the most disturbing conclusion: *American hospitals are far from safe.* Of the 1,047 patients, mistakes occurred in 480, or some 45 percent. Of those, almost 18 percent—one in six—experienced serious complications ranging from temporary disabilities to death. That result, incidentally, is amazingly similar to the Schimmel Yale–New Haven study done thirty years before.

Patients who were the victims of improper care suffered an average of four errors. One patient was victimized with fifty-two mistakes, the last of which killed him.

In several cases, lack of communication between departments and staff—a common failing of American hospitals—created the chaos:

- The purchasing department of the hospital ordered a new kind of tracheotomy tube, but failed to tell the nursing staff that it was calibrated differently from the old one. The nurse inserted the tube too far, killing the patient.
- As one shift of residents in the Intensive Care Unit gave way to another, they forget to remind the new shift that one of the patients was severely allergic to a certain drug, which they then dispensed to him.
- A patient was severely injured on the operating table, not because of a slip of the knife, but because the surgeon had been advised of the wrong course of action.

Covering Up Errors

Is there a conspiracy of silence that covers up daily errors in hospitals? Is there a purposeful ignorance that could explain why the Harvard study showed "safe hospitals," while this and other on-the-spot reports showed danger regularly lurking in the wards?

The answer is definitely yes.

Professor Andrews blows the whistle on the "gentlemanly" medical tradition that efficiently hides the truth:

"We were in training sessions for residents where they were told by attendings [staff doctors] to absolutely never fill out an occurrence report—that nurses do that. Or someone was improperly treated for a particular disorder and needed surgery as a result, but the surgeon wouldn't talk to the internal medicine people about the mistake because that might ruin their referrals. There's this culture of not being gentlemanly if you mention these problems."

One frightening aspect of the study showed that the longer the patients stayed in the hospital, the greater the chance that they would suffer damage. In fact, each day increased their chances of being damaged by six percent. (Some might wonder if these discouraging results were the reason researchers had to go to Britain to publish their study.)

The cause of these incidents of adverse care covered every aspect of medicine, including:

- Failure to order proper diagnostic tests
- Inadequate prep of the patient for surgery
- Surgery done when not indicated
- Improper dosage and monitoring of anesthesia
- Delay in undertaking treatment.
- Failure to provide patient with ordered drugs
- Wrong placement of drainage tubes
- Not taking proper antisepsis steps
- Patient's chart not properly updated
- Failure to properly communicate with the patient

What can we make of it all? If these figures are correct—and there's no reason to suspect otherwise, since they confirm earlier studies except for the flawed one from Harvard—then of the 31 million patients now admitted to hospitals annually, over 5 million will suffer a serious uneeded "episode" that will make them sicker. Upward of 500,000 will die as a result.

False Medical Records

Then why was the Harvard report so sanguine?

The answer, Dr. Andrews believes, is that most errors are not reported in the medical records. The obvious reason is professional defensiveness which masks the truth. *Of the 480 patients in the Chicago report who suffered iatrogenic damage, for example, only 113 of the incidents were ever entered on the medical records, and most of those involved less serious errors.*

But if hospitals know these facts, which have finally been confirmed several times, why don't they take remedial action with great fervor?

One reason is the desire not to accept the truth. It is hard for medical personnel to assume that the *routine* operation of the hospital is not intrinsically safe enough. That would mean herculean efforts had to be made each day, each hour, each minute, to protect the patients. To accept that one fact, which is apparently the truth, health providers would have to be ever alert, even anxious and tense—states of mind they prefer to ignore.

"We've led ourselves into thinking that errors are infrequent," Professor Andrews says, "so we don't incorporate the potential for error as part of the ongoing process." To correct that, she points out, would require a different hospital environment, one that is not *defensive* and in which mistakes are first openly discussed, then carefully documented in writing. "Of course," she adds, "that's easier said than done."

Obviously, the television world of medicine is preferable to the less sanguine world of reality.

A recent study conducted by Dr. Sanford E. Feldman of the University of California–Mt. Zion Medical Center shows how complacency, carelessness, and inattention to detail can together create a killing machine in our hospitals.

Dr. Feldman details eight cases of mistakes—sloppy medical care that is all too frequent—that led to the death of all but one patient.

The damning incidents, four of which follow, cover the full spectrum of hospital care.

- A woman was admitted to the hospital for surgery to correct an aneurysm in her abdomen. The anesthesiologist asked that a prepared and labeled unit of blood be brought in—just in case. The nurse returned with the blood, signing that it was for this patient. The doctor didn't check that the blood was correct. He infused into the patient, but after 100 cc, it became clear that something was wrong. The patient suffered intractable bleeding and died. The blood had been labeled for another patient, but no one had noticed.

- An older man was admitted to the hospital from a nursing home in a comatose state. Even though he was known to be diabetic, he was given glucose intravenously in the ambulance. The first night, a specialist wrote orders for "twenty units of regular insulin with each cc of IV fluids." The next day, the patient was not visited by any physician, and by the following day he was in a coma.

  He was suffering from a profound hypoglycemic condition with a low blood sugar count of only 18 (70 to 110 is normal). He died five days later. The medical record claimed he died of "pneumonia, congestive failure, organic brain syndrome." There was not a word about preventable hypoglycemia.

- A man was admitted for elective cataract surgery. He had a past history of pulmonary disease and high blood pressure. Two months before, glaucoma surgery was canceled when he had respiratory collapse after the administration of two local anesthestics, Lidocaine and Marcaine.

Now, once again, the patient was mistakenly prepared for his cataract operation with the same local anesthetics. He went into immediate respiratory collapse and needed intubation and oxygen support to be revived. Surgery was discontinued, but three days later an electrocardiogram showed that he had suffered a heart attack. He then suffered urinary retention and a subpubic operation was decided upon. Again he was given a local anesthetic—Xylocaine—resulting in another respiratory failure and cardiac arrest. He died three weeks later. His medical record included a warning note that local anesthesia should not have been used.

- A forty-nine-year-old man was given arthroscopic surgery to repair a right knee. The instrument was a CO_2 laser. The leasing company supplied a technician to handle the gas laser. But for some reason, the leasing company had moved the position of the pressure release valve. Not knowing this, and seeking stronger gas infusion, the technician released a blast of CO_2 with enough pressure to inflate a truck tire. The gas pushed past the knee joint, the tourniquet, and into the chest cavity, where it compressed the patient's heart and lungs. The patient suffered permanent brain damage.

Medical Cover-Ups?

One key problem in iatrogenic death is that hospitals tend not to report the incidents accurately. Either they have no effective system to monitor the damage or they are engaged in a medical cover-up. In either case, the extent of the damage is unknown and cannot be faced and improved.

A probe of hospitals by New York City showed that

many are less than candid about what went wrong. St. Vincent's Hospital in Manhattan, for example, reported to the state only two cases of "adverse incidents" in an entire year, which is ludicrous. On the other hand, Montefiore Medical Center in the Bronx admitted to 469 such incidents.

Increasingly, New York City and state authorities are trying to reduce poor care by inspecting hospitals for egregious cases of medical error. One prominent case involved Jonathan Larson, the author of the Pulitzer Prize–winning musical *Rent*, who died after visiting two hospital emergency rooms.

After dinner and rehearsal the Sunday before the opening, he suddenly complained of chest pains, dizziness, and difficulty in breathing. He was taken by ambulance to the Cabrini Medical Center emergency room, where they took an X ray and an electrocardiogram, both of which seemed normal. The doctor wrote "no cardiac disease." The pain was attributed to stress or even food poisoning. They pumped his stomach, gave him charcoal to absorb any toxins, and sent him home.

The next day he rested and felt somewhat better. On Tuesday, he suddenly took sick again and was taken to St. Vincent Hospital's emergency room where he told a nurse that on a scale of ten, his chest pain would be seven. She classified his case as urgent but didn't speak to a doctor about the vital sign readings.

The next day, the emergency room physician gave him another chest X ray and an electrocardiogram, which were also interpreted as normal. He was diagnosed as having a viral syndrome and was discharged as improved. On the cab ride home, Larson again complained of pain in his chest. At the hospital the next day a cardiologist read the electrocardiogram and indicated a possible myocardial infarction, a heart attack. But apparently there was no follow-up.

That night, Larson's play opened. The following morning, after an interview with the *New York Times*, he returned home. At 3:30, his roommate arrived home and found Larson lying on the kitchen floor, dead.

An autopsy showed the cause of death as an "aortic dissection due to cystic medial degeneration of unknown etiology." There was a foot-long tear in the aorta, the body's main blood vessel.

State health officials concluded that both hospitals were guilty of omissions and errors. While the state admitted that diagnosis of such a tear is difficult, they found that neither of the hospitals' diagnoses were correct. Further tests, they felt, should have been made. The hospitals were fined by the state and the relatives are contemplating a malpractice suit.

Another sudden death of a young person prompted a further probe, this time of the work of residents in training. In March 1998, state inspectors—doctors, nurses, and auditors—swept down without warning on twelve New York hospitals to check out whether young residents were being properly supervised by superiors or overworked in violation of state laws designed to protect patients. The surprise raids were designed to keep the hospitals from stage-managing the inspection. Not only is that a common defensive measure, but special firms work with hospitals to prepare them for inspections, which can help hospitals conceal their shortcomings.

The state regulatory probes began after the death of eighteen-year-old Libby Zion, daughter of a prominent journalist, when she was admitted to New York Hospital–Cornell Medical Center with a high fever. A grand jury found that the overworked, relatively unsupervised doctors in training contributed to her death. An appeals court exonerated the doctors, but the incident led to new state laws regarding the training of hospital residents.

The *New York Times* interviewed several residents who admitted they worked longer hours than the law allowed (eighty hours per week). They also confessed that they made diagnoses and started treatments on patients without the guidance of senior physicians, which is illegal.

One resident described how he worked 118.5 hours

the previous week, which was a typical load. Because of fatigue, he said, "you tend to miss things. You let things fall through the cracks that can come back to bite you."

He also lamented the lack of training from senior doctors. "My education was supposed to continue during residency and it barely is."

New York state investigators detailed several cases where lack of supervision of hospital residents resulted in injury or death. At Long Island Jewish a patient was given the wrong medication because of "inadequate resident supervision." A patient at St. Barnabas with a hand problem who developed an infection and died was cared for by residents and never seen by the attending physician. At Mary Immaculate a resident who "was not effectively supervised" prematurely removed a breathing tube, causing respiratory arrest. At New York Methodist, ten of eleven charts in the pediatric unit showed no evidence that the residents handling the care had been supervised.

The lack of supervision of hospital trainees often reaches tragic, or ridiculous, proportions. At the world-renowned Columbia Presbyterian Hospital in New York City, residents were recently discovered conducting a large-scale illegal practice in plastic surgery. Two renegade residents admitted to doing up to 136 illegal operations, including liposuction, all alone without a nurse or supervising doctor.

The state health department report explains that patients heard about the cut-rate surgery by word of mouth, then contacted the residents on their beepers. On weekends and early in the morning when the attending physicians were absent, they were taken into empty offices for surgery.

The scandal came to the surface when one of the residents, Dr. James Brady, did a secret $700 liposuction on a hairdresser who suffered a post-operative infection. A doctor at New York Hospital who treated the infection blew the whistle. The result was that Columbia was fined $66,000 for 36 different violations.

Quite a bit of cash was taken in, but the residents

claim they never took any personally. Supposedly it all went into a fund for medical conventions. The most surprising aspect of the stealth surgery was that it was an "open secret" at the hospital. "It was known to people" who hushed it up, says Dr. Barbara DeBuono, state health commissioner.

Can Hospital Damage Be Prevented?

How much of the daily damage done in our hospitals is preventable, and how much is just the necessary dark side of modern medicine that we have to accept?

Prominent researchers have tackled that sensitive question of "preventable" and "unpreventable" hospital deaths. At the Rand Corporation, Drs. R. W. Dubois and R. H. Brook conducted a study entitled "Preventable Deaths: Who, How Often, and Why?" which they published in the *Annals of Internal Medicine.*

They studied twelve hospitals, where Medicare inpatients had a death rate of 6.5 percent. One sixth to one-fourth (16 to 25 percent) of these deaths were judged to be "preventable" with the correct care.

The simplest mistakes in the hospital can not only be deadly, but equally important, they can happen in the "best" of institutions.

At the Dana-Farber Cancer Institute in Boston, a hospital of the highest repute, one of the patients was Betsy Lehman, who was not only an award-winning health columnist for the *Boston Globe,* but her husband was a scientist on the hospital staff.

The thirty-nine-year-old woman was suffering from breast cancer and nearing the end of a three-month chemotherapy treatment. She was on a drug called cyclophoshamide, plus another drug to shield her from the excessive side effects of chemotherapy. All was going well until one day she started to get worse, a condition that became more serious each day. Finally she died.

Of breast cancer? No. Of an overdose of chemotherapy. The maximum safe dosage is considered to be seven grams of cyclophoshamide. But in four days Ms. Lehman was given twenty-six grams of the toxic drug, which caused her heart to fail. The other drug was also dispensed at four times the correct dosage. During that time, irregularities in her heartbeat and abnormal lab results were ostensibly overlooked. At least a dozen doctors, nurses, and pharamacists missed the error, leading to her death.

She was not the only one victimized by the hospital's tragic mistake. The next day, at the same prestigious hospital, a fifty-two-year-old woman received a chemotherapy overdose and was rushed into intensive care. She survived, but suffered serious heart damage.

"If this can happen at a place like Dana-Farber . . . what is happening in other places?" asks Dr. O. Michael Colvin, director of the Duke University Comprehensive Cancer Center.

Dangerous Drug Reactions

Apparently, much the same thing, if not worse. Adverse drug reactions are among the leading killers in hospitals, where billions of doses are administered each year, many of them incorrectly.

In an Annapolis, Maryland, hospital, the night shift pharmacist received a call from a nurse. They had run out of heparin, a blood thinner used to flush out IVs. The pharmacist opened the refrigerator and grabbed a bottle to fill several syringes with the medicine. But instead of heparin, the pharmacist grabbed a bottle of morphine, which was soon coursing through the body of three sick infants. Fortunately, the babies survived. What had happened was that the pharmacist had picked up the wrong bottle, which was beside the other, one of the common mistakes in dealing with thousands of modern drugs.

To learn how often the wrong drug, or the wrong dose, was given to patients, a rigorous study was recently done on 4,031 adult patients in two major hospitals. The goal was to find the frequency of ADEs (Adverse Drug Events) and how many people they injured or killed.

The hospitals were among the most highly respected in the nation, Massachusetts General Hospital and the Brigham and Women's Hospital, both in Boston. The patients were *all* those admitted to eleven units of the hospitals over a six-month period from February through July 1993. (The study was published in 1995.)

The study's two leading researchers, Dr. David Bates of Brigham and Dr. Lucian Leape of the Harvard School of Public Health, found that the drug damage rate proved to be quite high—247 ADEs and 194 potential ADEs, affecting one in sixteen patients. Extrapolated out for the year, it means that 3,800 patients in those two hospitals would face drug damage.

Three patients died from the ADEs, representing one percent of all those affected. That would mean thirty-eight deaths a year from drug events just in those two hospitals, no small tally considering we are dealing with only two of 6,200 hospitals—and two of the best at that. In addition, twelve percent of the ADEs were *life-threatening* and thirty percent were "serious."

As an example of a serious or life-threatening drug event, they describe a patient with "first degree atrioventricular block who received a beta-blocker and developed complete heart block requiring temporary pacing." An example of a "potential" problem was "a patient who received penicillin despite a known allergy to penicillin, but did not react." What in common parlance would be called a therapeutic "narrow escape."

Using these careful study results by leading researchers, we could extrapolate them to mean that among the 31 million hospital patients a year nationwide, some 2 million will suffer ADEs.

We can therefore count on some 20,000 deaths nationwide from "Adverse Drug Events" this year. Making the picture even bleaker, if that's possible, we have to add almost a quarter of a million "life-threatening" incidents from the medicines pre-scribed for hospital patients by their physicians.

Medication errors are particularly frequent and serious among the aged. A survey of nursing home pharmacies by the inspector general of HHS found that almost half the pharmacists believed that the patients are regularly given improper prescriptions, often with serious consequences.

The report includes audits of several Texas nursing homes where 17 percent—one in six—patients received "inappropriate" drugs, meaning that they were not rec-ommended for the elderly, or being used for illnesses they were not designed to treat, or they were medications not dispensed according to the doctor's prescription.

The result of these medication mistakes—most often involving pain-killing narcotics, anti-inflammatories and drugs for gastrointestinal ailments—were such numerous adverse reactions as falls and delirium.

This epidemic of mayhem can be costly not only in death, disability, and pain, but in money as well. The au-thors estimate that each ADE costs the hospital an addi-tional $2,000, not counting the malpractice costs or the injury to the patient. Most important, they learned that forty-two percent of the life-threatening and serious acci-dents were "preventable"—if hospitals learned why they were taking place and put in systems to head them off.

As a result of the discouraging results, Brigham and Women's Hospital has installed a new computerized sys-tem that they expect will cut down on errors. When the doctor, for instance, places a drug order, the computer scans the patient's record to see if he is already receiving an incompatible prescription. The hospital expects that the new system will cut out eighty-five percent of ordering errors and half of all drug injuries. Co-author of the study, Dr. Leape, believes (or hopes) that in a decade there will be a drug terminal alongside each patient's bed.

Medication errors are equally common in the hospi-tal's outpatient clinics. In fact, as that patient load increases rapidly, errors are even *more likely* to occur there than on hospital wards.

Sociologist David Phillips of the University of California, San Diego, a morbidity expert, has just completed a study showing that the outpatient clinic is a perfect setting for iatrogenic episodes caused by medication errors, in both the type of prescriptions and their dosage.

In the decade from 1983 to 1993, for instance, he and his team found that outpatient hospital visits for medical care increased by seventy-five percent. With this new traffic has come a large increase in medication errors and deaths.

Publishing in *Lancet*, Phillips explains that by 1993 one out of every 131 outpatient deaths was caused by medication errors—*a fourfold increase in drug mistakes per patient from 1983*. Was it due to the increased volume of prescriptions? No, that number went up only 1.4 times.

"Our data suggest," Phillips says, "that medical personnel may need to compensate for changes in medical care by increased vigilance in the delivery and monitoring of medication, especially for outpatients. There is growing concern about the quality and continuity of physician-patient relationships; in the case of medication errors, this concern may be justified."

The message should now be clear: the hospital, including its outpatient clinics, are susceptible to error of every nature, often at a frightening rate.

The Threat from Medications

An even graver threat to hospitalized patients than errors made in medications is the drugs themselves, even when they are supposedly properly prescribed by physicians.

A study published in JAMA *in April 1998 shocked the public with its conclusion that over 100,000 Americans die each year in hospitals from adverse drug reactions, or what is popularly known as dangerous "side effects."*

Bruce Pomeranz, a professor at the University of Toronto and co-author of the report, states that the problem is widespread in hospitals of all types and goes undetected because the FDA relies on those very hospitals, doctors, and pharmaceutical firms to report to them voluntarily, rather than seek out the information themselves. The FDA's numbers for hospital deaths due to adverse drug reactions, he says, are "absurdly low."

Pomeranz did no original research, but instead correlated thirty-nine previous studies on hospital medication deaths made over a period of thirty years and came up with his startling statistics. He found that seven percent of hospital patients, or 2.3 million cases, suffer adverse drug reactions. He excluded drug mistakes, drug abuse, and suicide, but included both prescription drugs and over-the-counter medicines either prescribed or recommended by the doctors.

The report created such turmoil in the medical community that Dr. David Bates of the Harvard Medical School—who, as we have seen, has conducted his own study of adverse reactions—attacked Pomeranz's study in an editorial in *JAMA*. "I think their estimates are probably high," he says. But he does admit that his own lower estimate is shocking nonetheless. Dr. Bates puts the toll from hospital drug reactions at closer to 50,000 deaths a year.

Bates concurs that the problem has been mainly overlooked by both doctors and hospitals. "It is a serious issue, and one that hasn't received the attention it deserves."

Who is to blame?

Dr. Bates places that mainly on the hospitals. "Hospitals should be more vigilant, because it is only at the hospital level that you can build an effective tracking system." That safeguard is something few institutions now have.

But, as is often the case, doctors have escaped much of the blame that truly belongs to them. Too often they rely on pharmaceutical manufacturers' salesmen ("detail men") for their information on medications, and are insufficiently aware of the complex side effects of the drugs they prescribe. Warnings regularly appear in medical journals when suspicious adverse reactions are reported. But too many doctors are not studious enough to keep track of them.

The result? Widespread death from medication.

Deadly Hospital Infections

Danger is obviously omnipresent in America's hospitals, in its wards and in its operating suites. One of the gravest threats to life and limb is picking up an infection—a commonplace hospital event that shows little sign of abetting. The Centers for Disease Control and Prevention (CDC) of the U.S. Public Health Service monitors the rate of hospital infections, which seems to be a stubborn and unyielding enemy.

"Nosocomial [hospital-acquired] infections are a major source of morbidity and mortality, affecting more than two million patients annually in the United States," say officials of the Hospital Infections Program of the CDC.

This is borne out by the awesome, almost unbelievable numbers of hospital deaths involved. The annual death toll at last count was 19,027 lives lost *outright*, plus the equally frightening tally of 58,092 "deaths to which infections contributed." This represents a scourge of almost 80,000 lives every year. Adding to the tally is the unpleasant fact that according to a study done by Dr. William R. Jarvis for the CDC, the rate of hospital infection rose thirty-six percent from 1975 to 1995 *despite* the smaller number of patients—37.7 million versus 35.9 million.

The cost of these two million infections is enormous in sickness, death, time, and money. The typical infection adds four extra days to the hospitalization at a cost of $2,100 more—or over $4 billion a year. (The urinary infections only added one day to the hospital stay, but in the case of a surgical infection, the stay was an extra full week.)

Worse yet, these numbers *do not* include infections following surgery in outpatient facilities, which is increasingly the site of operations. Nor does it include infections that show themselves after discharge from the hospital, which are generally not studied.

So as not to contaminate the study, the CDC authors dealt only with cases "for which there is no evidence that the infection was present or incubating at the time of hospital admission."

The Most Common Hospital Infections

Of all the infections reported in their study, the most common were urinary tract infections (UTI), followed by pneumonia, then by surgical site infections (SSI), and primary bloodstream infections (BSI). There were also infections in bones and joints, and central nervous and cardiovascular systems.

Did it make any difference what kind of hospital was involved?

Apparently not. The frequency of infections in hospitals was approximately the same whether the hospitals were large or small, community hospitals or major medical school institutions.

Surgery represents the gravest danger. In fact, the rate of infection in that field has not decreased in a decade. As the CDC points out. "SSI [surgical site infections] are a major infection control concern because they are associated with serious morbidity and high cost." Patients who undergo an operation also have higher rates of infection at other sites, such as pneumonia, UTI, and BSI.

The risk comes from bacteria in the operative field, the duration of the operation, plus, says the CDC, "the use of high risk devices such as ventilators, urinary catheters, and central intravascular lines during surgery and in the postoperative period."

The CDC report, which was published in *Clinical Microbiology Reviews*, lists twenty-five bacteria that invade the body in the hospital. But of those, certain "bugs" are responsible for the majority of the infections, especially the deadly ones. They include:

Escherichia coli (E. coli)
Staphlococcus aureus ("staph")
CoNS
Enterococcus spp.
Pseudomonas aeruginosa

When pneumonia was picked up in the hospital, staph and pseudomonas were the major agents, along with enterobacter spp.

Antibiotics Can Actually Create Infections

Antibiotics can, of course, cure many bacterial infections, but at the same time, their overuse helps *create* hospital infections. This extraordinary boon to man has its own iatrogenic side effect.

Almost one-third of all patients in our hospitals are on some form of antibiotic therapy. "However," warns the CDC authors, "it has become abundantly clear that the major nosocomial [in hospital] pathogens either are naturally resistant to clinically useful antimicrobial agents or possess the ability to acquire resistance."

Staphylococcus infections can create havoc in the hospital setting. They are responsible for pneumonia, surgical wound infections, and bloodstream infections. At one time the bug was vulnerable to attack by the methicillin group of antibiotics, which include methicillin, and the related oxacillin and nafcillin. Unfortunately, their widespread use has created staph germs that have developed resistance. In fact, the percentage of such resistance rose from a minor 2.4 percent in 1975 to 32 percent in 1992, and continues to rise.

In fact, 70 percent of hospital infections are due to microbes resistant to one or more antibioties. In 30 to 40 percent of the infections, the microbes are resistant to the first-line drug of choice.

The Growing Immunity to Vancomycin

Then came the supposed "silver bullet" against staph. It was an antibiotic called vancomycin, which saved many lives that would otherwise be lost. But now the clever staph germ has found ways to outwit man and is beginning to develop resistance to that antiobiotic as well— fighting desperately to block our battle against pathogens.

The latest CDC report tells of a new strain of staph that seems to be developing resistance to vancomycin. The first case, in 1996, involved a Japanese infant who developed staph from a boil after heart surgery. The infection showed "an intermediate resistance" to vancomycin, one step away from immunity.

Now that bug has shown up in the United States. In July 1997 a patient in Michigan developed a staph infection from the strain in a catheter used in kidney dialysis. He is now being treated by a combination of drugs that they hope will work.

"We were concerned it would emerge here," the CDC says. "It has emerged here, and we are concerned we're going to see it pop up in more places."

But the fight continues as drug companies develop new antibiotics to outwit the clever hospital staph bacteria. A new one called Synercid, developed by Rhone-Poulenc Rorer, killed the staph in the Japanese infant, and in the lab has shown to be effective in the Michigan case.

But despite the valiant efforts of scientists, infections continue to kill hospital patients every day. Everything in a hospital seems to conspire to create infections. It comes from the air, the water, the food, the blankets, the medical equipment. The air can transmit tuberculosis and Legionnaire's disease. When instruments are not fully sterilized, there is also the danger of infection, as with the loose handling of needles, scalpels, etc. And in the final analysis, a breakdown in old-fashioned personal hygiene by medical workers breeds staph.

Failure to Wash Hands

"The patient care staff," warn the authors, "must not forget the critical role of hand-washing."

Even though 150 years ago Dr. Ignaz Semmelweis, in Hungary, proved that hand-washing could prevent many infections—the unwashed hands of American hospital personnel still present one of the gravest dangers in an American hospital.

In Boston, an outbreak of a yeast infection was traced to medical staff workers who did not wash their hands after playing with their dogs. The infection made fifteen babies sick at Dartmouth–Hitchcock Medical Center in Lebanon, New Hampshire. One or two of the babies first became infected, then the doctors and nurses spread the disease to the others when they touched them.

Dr. William Jarvis of the Centers for Disease Control and Prevention, who investigated the case, explained that scrubbing is critical, especially when dealing with babies, whose immune systems are not fully developed. Perhaps the gravest problem is that health care workers either lie or are self-delusional. At that hospital, two-thirds of those questioned said they *always* scrubbed between patients. But when they were secretly observed, it turned out that they only washed between patients one-third of the time.

No one died in that outbreak, but infants at the Children's Hospital in Boston were less lucky. Four infants in the neonatal intensive care unit died of a bacterial infection in the summer of 1997 when they were stricken with *pseudomonas aeruginosa*. Usually easily curable in adults, the bacteria can cause a fatal blood infection in those with weak immune systems, as in premature infants.

One infant became infected with it and recovered, but the bacterium was passed, probably on the hands of employees, to the other babies. In September 1997, the hospi-

tal closed the unit temporarily and started to take
infection control seriously. They examined all the equipment in the ward for the bacteria and have now—only
after the deaths—insisted that workers wash their hands
with two types of antibacterial soap.

The hand-washing problem is so serious that at Cook
County Hospital in Chicago, guards were stationed to remind doctors, nurses, and others to wash their hands—
and to prevent surgeons from leaving the operating room
in their possibly infected scrub suits.

Such precautions are important, but in a way it is almost pitiful to discover that trained medical personnel
don't know, or don't care, about the harm to patients that
can result from those invisible little "bugs."

*The tragic aspect of the 20,000 to 80,000 deaths a year from
hospital infections is that despite all modern technology and
knowledge, it persists. And despite the high death toll, hospitals
in America have done very little to improve the situation.*

Can the hospital infection epidemic be prevented?
Much of it can, *if* hospitals are scrupulous in following
the guidelines set up for an infection surveillance and control program.

The CDC learned that infections could be cut down
thirty-two percent—which would save up to 25,000 lives
a year—*if* hospitals followed all their guidelines. These
suggestions include having a full-time infection control
practitioner for each 250 beds, along with a hospital epide-
miologist. To fight surgical wound infections, feedback of
the infection rates to the surgeons is essential so that he
can face the problem better the next time.

Hospitals Ignore Anti-Infection Regimen

Has this been done in most hospitals?

The CDC has set up a system for studying how well
their guidelines are being put into practice. Their conclusion is less than optimistic. In fact it is downright discouraging. *Their study indicates that only one in fifty hospitals*

fully carries out the necessary anti-infection routines. The prevention rate is only between six and nine percent, leaving up to 94 percent of the deadly risk intact.

Since there's not much difference among hospitals when it comes to iatrogenic disease, drug mistakes, unwanted events, and infections, then why choose one hospital over another?

If hospitals seem about the same in *negative* terms, the same is not true in a positive sense. There are exceptions, but by and large the profession looks to the university teaching centers—from Mt. Sinai in New York to UCLA University Hospital in Los Angeles—which are noted for their *positive* performance.

Hospitals directly affiliated with medical schools do the most research and strive to practice the purest medicine regardless of the patient's pocketbook or the economic incentive of the doctors. At Yale–New Haven Hospital, for example, the salaried physicians in the faculty medical practice generally do not earn any additional money for their treatment of patients.

All Hospitals Are Not Created Equal

Obviously there are differences in the performance of hospitals, and New York State is in the midst of an unprecedented study to check into the quality of care in the state's major institutions. Under the guidance of former state health commissioner, Dr. Mark Chassins, who is now at Mt. Sinai, they have put together an annual survey of the *survival rate* of patients undergoing two major operations—cardiac bypass and angioplasty—at hospitals throughout the state.

The survey is unprecedented, because doctors and hospitals have long fought what is usual in consumer affairs: being graded and having the information given out freely to the public. The myth is that patients should be willing to go to any hospital with the secure belief that they will come out alive and cured.

This survey shows quite the opposite—that there are large differences in performance from one hospital to another in these common operations (half a million heart bypass surgeries a year) that the educated patient should know about.

Called "Coronary Artery Bypass Surgery in New York State, 1993–1995," the study was issued by that state's Department of Health in August 1997. It measured the survival rate of the operation in thirty-one hospitals, from New York City to Buffalo.

To ensure a level playing field, the figures were all risk-weighted. That is, a hospital that handled the most severe cases would not be penalized, nor would those with the easiest cases be rewarded. An eighty-year-old man with a chronic heart condition cannot be compared to a forty-year-old patient who has just experienced his first heart problem.

Coronary bypass surgery is a procedure in which a vein or an artery from another part of the body is used to create an alternate path for blood to flow to the heart, bypassing the problem—which is an arterial blockage of plaque on the artery wall. Typically, a section of one of the large veins in the leg, the radial artery in the arm or the mammary artery in the chest, is used to construct the bypass.

One or more bypasses may be performed during a single operation, since providing several routes for the blood supply to travel is believed to improve long-term success. Triple and quadruple, even quintuple, bypasses are often done for this reason and not necessarily because the patient's condition is more severe.

Of the 19,283 cases studied in New York State, there were 485 deaths, for an average mortality of 2.52 percent. But the rate among the hospitals varied greatly.

The winner? St. Joseph's Hospital in Syracuse, New York, with a risk-adjusted mortality rate just slightly above *one* percent, actually 1.16.

The loser? Bellevue Hospital in New York City, whose RAMR (Risk Ajusted Mortality Rate) was a scary 5.67 percent.

Most hospitals sat alongside the average line, with a few other near-stars such as Ellis Hospital (Schenactady), North Shore (Manhasset), and United Health Services (Binghamton). The near-losers included Millard Fillmore (Buffalo), St. Luke's Roosevelt (New York City), and Upstate Medical Center (Albany).

Grading the Heart Surgeons

Perhaps the most startling aspect of the study was that they rated surgeons as well. It was done by name, something the profession has fought against since time immemorial. To doctors, being graded is a frightening thought. It could give consumers the upper hand in choosing their own physicians, rather than leaving it to chance.

Who were the most successful surgeons? In this case, those with the highest survival rate for patients. The winners were Dr. M. Marvisti at St. Joseph's, with only one death among 431 heart bypass surgeries, for an adjusted survival rate of 99.7 percent, and Dr. E. Bennett at Albany Medical Center, with one death out of 281 cases, for an adjusted survival rate of 99.61 percent.

Others with less than one percent mortality were Dr. Sarabu at Westchester County Medical Center, 99.48; L. Durban at St. Francis Hospital, 99.46; Dal, Col. R., at St. Peter's, 99.21; T. Canavan at Albany Medical Center Hospital, 99.07; A. Nazem at St. Joseph's, and W. Scott at Winthrop–University Hospital, 99.01.

When the state rated doctors doing bypass operations at more than one institution, a few additional names with high survival rates appeared at about the 99 percent riskadjusted survival level. They included T. Canavan from Albany and Ellis; A. Culliford at NYU Medical Center; and J. McIlduff at Ellis and St. Peter's.

(A copy of the report can be obtained from the Health Department in Albany.)

A second report has now been issued, one on angioplasty operations. Angioplasty is a technique in which a balloon is placed into the blocked artery with a catheter, then inflated, pushing out the harmful plaque. The study showed an overall mortality rate of less than one percent (.09) with 194 deaths in 21,707 operations.

Here, surprisingly, the winners were Bellevue (which fared the worst in bypasses), Buffalo General, Montefiore-Moses (New York City), North Shore (Manhasset), Presbyterian (New York City), St. Francis (Beacon), and St. Peter's (Albany), all of which had risk-adjusted mortality of less than a half percent. Bellevue and Buffalo General had no deaths at all, in a total of 654 cases.

The losers, with mortality at 1.5 percent and up, included Albany Medical Center, Beth Israel (New York City), Long Island Jewish (Nassau County), Montefiore-Weiler (New York City), Strong Memorial (Rochester), and Upstate Medical Center (Albany). The most angioplasties were done by St. Francis, a total of 2,114 with only nine deaths.

The other high volume angioplasties done at hospitals were 1,498 at Lenox Hill, with 24 deaths; 1,464 at North Shore, with 8 deaths; 1,497 at Rochester General with 12 deaths; 1,078 at St. Joseph's with 10 deaths; and 1,025 at Westchester County Medical Center, with 8 deaths.

The differences shown in the New York State report are illuminating because almost never are specific hospitals measured for quality. However, there is an increase in the number of studies of care in *unnamed* hospitals, and much of it is discouraging.

Washington Gets Involved

The federal government, which spends some forty percent of the entire trillion-dollar health bill, is trying to gauge how well their money is spent. The government launched the Health Care Quality Improvement Initiative to check on how well hospitals were handling various illnesses. As part of that program, they put together a giant study of all Acute Myocardial Infarction (AMI) heart attack cases involving Medicare patients in four states: Connecticut, Iowa, Wisconsin, and Alabama.

In all, 14,108 prime hospitalizations due to these heart attacks were studied. A panel of doctors examined the medical records and tried to compare the *actual* treatment in hospitals with guidelines on care compiled by the American College of Cardiology and the American Heart Association.

How well did the hospitals do? Apparently, not too well. Perhaps even worse.

The doctors found the following:

- Thirteen percent of the patients—about 1,800— probably did not have an acute myocardial infarction to begin with.
- Among the "ideal" candidates for treatment, less than half received beta-blockers, which reduce the demand for oxygen and cut down heart attacks and sudden death. And among that same group, a quarter did not receive nitroglycerin for chest pain.
- About thirty percent did not receive heparin to avoid clots.
- Seventeen percent did not receive aspirin treatment.

Now that we know the potential dangers, the question is: Are there sufficient checks on what hospitals are doing or not doing?

Not really. The only industrywide screen is accreditation, a rather simple one that is accorded to almost all who apply. That is supervised by the Joint Commission on Accreditation of Health Plans, headquartered in Chicago.

The commission accredits 18,000 health care organizations including hospitals, health care plans and PPOs, home health services, nursing homes, and ambulatory care facilities including outpatient surgery centers, group practices, and clinical labs.

It is the only meaningful standard in the hospital business, so a good deal of attention is paid to it. It usually substitutes for both Medicare and Medicaid certification by the government. In many states, accreditation by the "Joint Commission," as it is generally known, fulfills the licensing requirements. They employ some five hundred surveyors—including doctors, nurses, health care administrators, pharmacists, social workers, etc.—who visit and check out the institutions.

Is it an honest checkup? Yes. Is it a thorough screen? Not really.

It performs all the customary and usual checks but *does not* do the kind of quality investigation we have witnessed at Yale–New Haven, Brigham, Massachusetts General, or the Chicago teaching hospital, where an enormous number of medical and pharmaceutical errors were uncovered and care was much worse than anyone had ever thought.

Various Forms of Accreditation

The accreditation, which covers 5,155 hospitals, comes in many categories, differentiated by quality. The top hospitals, some 620, have accreditation "With Commendation," including such teaching hospitals as Yale–New Haven. Approximately another 200 institutions are merely "Accredited." The bulk of the hospitals, about 4,200, are accredited "With Recommendations for Improvement." They are given a stipulated amount of time to carry out the improvements in order to become fully accredited.

(There are surprises in the list. Massachusetts General, long considered a top tier institution, is only accredited "With Recommendations for Improvement.")

About two hundred hospitals have failed the cutoff, and fall into one of four negative categories, including "Provisional Accreditation" (having failed the first survey, they are given a second chance six months later); "Conditional Accreditation," where they are given a specified amount of time to fix their problems; "Preliminary Non-Accreditation," which is the entry to the slippery slope of being "Non-Accredited" because of "significant noncompliance with Joint Commission Standards."

It can also mean that the hospital has voluntarily withdrawn from the whole process, which is itself a self-damning move.

Can you learn how your local hospital has been judged?

Yes. You can call Customer Service of the Joint Commission at 630-792-5800 and they will tell you what category your hospital is in. And you can request a full report on the hospital, most of which they now have on file. They will mail it to you free of charge. Or you can use the Internet, a new service of the organization.

The Internet steps are:

1. Type in www.jcaho.org
2. When their web page comes up, click "Health Care Organizations and Professionals" in the center. After that page loads, click "Quality Check" in the upper left. You will get a "Directory of Accreditation."
3. Scan left and double click "Search for Health Care Org."
4. Type in what type of organization—Hospital, Home Health Care, HMO, etc.—then follow the directions for state, name of hospital, city.
5. The screen will tell you the type of accreditation, and advise you on whether a report on the hospital is available for downloading.

Accreditation has progressed as a system, but it still lacks the stringent quality controls we have discussed here. So it should be considered a *rough* guide to your hospital, which is presumably better than nothing.

In New York City, Public Advocate Mark Green criticized the work of the Joint Commission in allegedly overlooking everything from poor patient care to sloppy record keeping in its work of judging New York City hospitals every three years. He pointed out that the hospitals were told when the Joint Commission inspections were to take place, enabling the hospitals to spruce up, even to hire extra doctors and staff.

Fictional Hospital Bills

One of the strangest aspects of the hospital situation in America is financial: the bills presented to patients on their discharge. The first anomaly is that they are extraordinarily high, much more than anyone could guess. The second fact is that the bills make absolutely no sense.

Stories of fifteen dollars for an aspirin are quite true, *mainly because the hospital bill really is a piece of fiction.* It is designed to allot to each patient not the true cost of his or her own care, but a portion of the total upkeep of the hospital!

A perfect example of inflated bills is one received by a patient at Yale–New Haven Hospital. He was admitted at midnight on an emergency basis because of blood in his urine. The patient was immediately put into a semiprivate room and a catheter placed in his bladder through the penis to drain the fluid. He spent that night in the hospital. The following day he was given a CAT scan for diagnosis of possible kidney cancer, which proved to be negative. There was no surgery and nothing else was done. The following morning—after only thirty-six hours in the hospital—he was discharged.

The care was excellent; the procedure the correct one.

The bill? One or two thousand dollars? Hardly. It was a startling $5,350, which the patient found laughable, if only because his insurance covered all but a few hundred dollars.

If the bill were honest, then Yale–New Haven couldn't make ends meet with its enormous overhead as a teaching hospital. Nor could it provide extensive charity service for the legions of poor in the area. In a way, it's a Catch-22 situation. We would like the bills to be honest, but then the hospital couldn't function at the elevated academic and medical level it does.

Third party insurers, whether Medicare or the HMOs, have undoubtedly raised the cost of hospital care, probably doubling it in real dollars over a generation. Medicare and Medicaid patients are not usually concerned about the inflated costs because Medicare has a one-time deductible of $760 no matter how large the bill. Medicaid bills are usually covered one hundred percent.

High Co-Payments for Some

But the billing inflation becomes a real problem when the patient has indemnity or HMO "freedom" insurance that requires a co-payment on hospital bills.

If the hospital is overcharging that patient by $3,000, then he must usually pay an extra $600, or twenty percent of the bill. But what of a patient who requires cancer surgery and chemotherapy and might be liable for $150,000 in treatment? Then he must come up with $30,000 of his own money in co-payment. Who can afford that? Then the once academic concern about inflated hospital bills becomes a harsh reality.

In the case of indemnity insurance, many companies check the care *retrospectively*, after it's completed. At that point they can—and sometimes do—refuse to pay for much of it, either because it is not "covered" or they claim it is not "medically necessary." The patient is then in a position of fighting his insurance company so as not to go bankrupt.

We will later look at the whole question of insurance and what to do about the forty million uninsured (See Chapter VIII).

The situation may even be worse. Hard-pressed hospitals have become harsh, both in hiring collection agencies to get their money and even by filing liens against home owners who haven't paid in full. It's an especially strong blow since patients who must personally pay part, or all, of the hospital bill suspect that the hospital has cheated them—which it probably has. The "fictional" bills were designed for third-party insurers, not for real people who have to pay real money.

In Connecticut, the state has set up a consumer information service to help patients who believe their hospital bills are unfair. The office tries to adjudicate large bills by dealing with the hospital and the insurance company, and points out that in eighteen months it has saved patients $200,000, actually a small amount considering it is statewide.

"We try to help people," says a state spokesperson, "but I make it clear that although the hospitals and insurers usually talk to me, they don't have to. They have no legal obligation to do anything about reducing their bills or raising their insurance coverage."

Since Connecticut has no public hospitals—or "for-profit" ones either—that would provide free care, they tax all hospitals a six percent sales tax on all bills, plus an $8\frac{1}{4}$ percent tax on "gross earnings," and use *part* of the money to subsidize free hospital care for those in need. They also point out that Yale–New Haven Hospital provides a great deal of free care, mainly because of their enormous endowment fund.

(This halfway measure in no way makes up for the need for free care, which is provided directly by public hospitals around the nation—hospitals that make up one in five of all institutions. New York City, for example, has eleven public hospitals, truly open to the public.)

The money crunch has reached crisis proportions in hospitals, many of which are going broke. The reasons are many: the high cost of medical technology; the lower HMO and Medicare and Medicaid payments; the reduction in the number of days a typical patient is hospitalized; and the drain of maintaining 35 to 40 percent empty beds.

Huckster Hospital Ads

To help fill those beds and fight the competition, hospitals throughout America are now embarked on lavish and near-desperate advertising campaigns in a struggle for survival.

Like toothpaste and soap makers, they trumpet their wares, sometimes in a huckster manner, advertising on radio and in full-page ads in such prestigious papers as the *New York Times*. Since Medicare patients and the indemnity insured have free choice of hospitals, each new patient, particularly the aged ones, can mean $10,000 or $25,000 or even $50,000, an added income to a cash-strapped institution.

Some ads trumpet their care, both its excellence and, in some cases, the newness of the technology. One of the most active in the New York area is the Staten Island University Hospital, which takes out regular radio ads describing their advanced procedures and potential cures, including radioactive techniques for brain tumors. North Shore University Hospital and the Long Island Jewish Hospital are included in large print ads for the "toasting" of the prostate gland, an outpatient procedure that uses microwave-catheter technology to reduce enlargement.

A recent advertisement in the *New York Times* congratulated the New York University Liver Transplant Center as being ranked number one on the East Coast. In the special issue of *New York* magazine highlighting the city's best doctors, the hospitals ran numerous ads side by side with photos of superior physicians, hoping the doctors' prestige would rub off on them. On the Op-Ed page of the *New York Times*, Mt. Sinai runs ads touting their reputation for good medicine to upper-income readers seeking superior care. Robert Wood Johnson Hospital in New Jersey has committed a near fortune in ads in the *New York Times* to let everyone know of its many awards.

Celebrity patients are often featured in ads. New York Hospital–Cornell told the story of how when Larry King feared a heart attack coming on, he flew medevac 3,000 miles from LA to the hospital, where he underwent an angioplasty and was back on TV a week later.

Hospitals Merge and Close

All this comes from the pressure to survive in an arena of closings, mergers, and acquisitions of hospitals, more than reminiscent of Wall Street. To save money, two of the most prestigious hospitals in the nation, New York Hospital (Cornell Medical Center) and Columbia University's Presbyterian Hospital have merged, as have many others.

Now with extensive use of psychochemicals, psychiatric hospitals are closing at a rapid rate. From 1970 to 1990 fourteen such institutions nationwide shut their doors. And the trend is accelerating. Just since 1990, thirty-two have closed and ten more are about to end their operation. On Long Island, four prominent psychiatric hospitals—Central Islip Psychiatric Center, Pilgrim State Psychiatric Center, Kings Park Psychiatric Center, and the Long Island Developmental Center—are closing. All the remaining patients, 1,300 in all, will be shifted to a remaining piece of Pilgrim State.

Nationwide, general hospitals are facing the same erosion. A study entitled "The Hospital Acquisition Report, Third Edition, 1997," explains that "during 1996, one hospital changed hands for each day of the year." The report adds: "The health care delivery system in the United States is undergoing tremendous and rapid change, primarily as a result of the increasing market penetration of managed care." Once again we see the footprints of the HMO bogeyman.

One of the strongest merger and buy-out movements of the past five years has been the consolidation of "for-profit," or money-making, privately owned hospitals. This has been happening concurrently with the acquisition of voluntary, community nonprofit hospitals by their peers and by for-profit hospitals, who like to call themselves "investor-owned."

In the last three years, one hundred struggling community hospitals have been taken over by hospital chains that can better handle the cutthroat competition for HMO contracts, which have become as important as government money.

Barbarians at the Medical Gates

The leader in this gobbling up, which often aggravates local people who miss their former community hospital, has been the giant Columbia-HCA Healthcare Corporation, which owns half of all the for-profit hospitals in America. Typically, the new for-profit owners cut costs, eliminate personnel, and try to make a buck where there was once a deficit.

Whether they practice quality medicine as well is an unanswered question. There are grave doubts about their dedication to research, the amount of charity care they provide, and whether they employ sufficient personnel and provide the latest, most expensive treatments to their patients.

Columbia-HCA has gotten into fiscal and ethical trouble, possibly as a result of its superaggressive campaign to take over more and more hospitals, both for-profit and community-based ones. Its technique is totally business-like, and comes in seven steps, which reportedly are:

1. Fill more beds than other hospitals, which they have done.
2. Bring in doctors as limited partners in the hospital so they can share in the profits and keep a financial eye on hospital treatments.
3. Give hospital managers profit goals and reward them with large bonuses if they meet them.
4. Cut the staff to save money. Columbia's hospitals employ seventeen percent less people than voluntary hospitals.
5. Charge more than other hospitals. In Columbia's case the average bill is $4,374 against $4,059 per patient elsewhere.
6. Push outpatient treatment instead of inpatient admissions, mainly because Medicare pays more generously for those services.
7. Bill the government for expensive treatments much more often than other hospitals.

The *New York Times* described a case of Columbia pressing their medical people to the limit to make profits. At the Michael Reese Hospital and Medical Center in Chicago, a hospital bought out by Columbia, the top executives of Columbia's Midwest division called a meeting in the hospital's board room to lambaste the fourteen department heads for not cutting costs aggressively enough.

The director of medicine at the time, Mark Singer, remembers that the Columbia brass focused on the case of three uninsured patients who had been sent to a special heart unit for treatment, chastising them for admitting such patients, who were called "self pays."

"My father owned and operated a millinery factory in the garment district," Mr. Singer says, "and I never witnessed such an extent of demeaning, debasing, and devaluing behavior in the tough street environment as I personally experienced then."

Forcing Out the Poor Patient

His ire is morally correct. Beyond that there is the immorality of Columbia-HCA turning away the uninsured, something that is less likely in voluntary hospitals, and almost never in public hospitals, who take care of charity cases regardless of who they are. If we continue to yield to for-profit medicine, we might as well throw Hippocrates out with the soiled bathwater.

Because of the federal investigation of Columbia-HCA, they have adopted several new policies, including a less aggressive public stance, less expansion, new management, using local hospital names rather then "Columbia," and the possible sale of one-third of their 350 for-profit hospital chain.

Public hospitals that do care for the poor are having a tough time of it, especially as HMOs, which are mainly for-profit, keep cutting their payments for hospitalization. MetroHealth Medical Center in Cleveland is the only major public hospital in the area, and must bear the brunt of Medicaid low-pay patients, as well as pure charity cases for which there is not compensation—everyone from poor working people to the homeless and AIDS patients. To keep their city hospital from being absorbed by a community or for-profit institution, they have fought to stay in business, working against the odds.

Their county subsidy was cut in half when the city investment fund lost money. They failed to renew a long-standing contract to provide care for Kaiser Permanente subscribers. They had to work with less Medicaid money as that program was converted into an HMO called Ohio-Care. Meanwhile, their costs went up for their medical teaching program, new technology, and outreach programs in poorer neighborhoods, including one that most hospitals avoid like the plague. They have a live-in program for addicted and alcoholic mothers, and have set up a clinic in an Hispanic neighborhood for maternal and pediatric services.

How did they stay alive? They started cutting out specialists and hiring more primary doctors, who are cheaper, if not better trained. They eliminated four hundred workers and plan to cut three hundred more. They set up a new price structure, including a sliding scale for baby deliveries based on the difficulty of the case. They have cut down the length of hospital stays. (Shades of HMOs.) Still, with all those economies, they still need $110 million a year in government subsidies to stay alive.

Keeping hospitals alive is the theme of twenty-first-century medicine, since the nation probably could eliminate 750 hospitals without feeling a health pinch—except for geographic distribution.

But how can they stay alive, considering the lowered payments from HMOs and the new reduced rates for Medicare and Medicaid that came from the so-called balanced budget deal of 1997?

The Drive to Attract Foreign Patients

One answer is to attract more patients. Advertising is one method. A second method is to bring in foreigners to fill all those empty beds. For years, wealthy foreigners seeking surgery beat a trail to our better hospitals. The president of the United Arab Emirates checked into the Mayo for neck surgery, bringing 140 people with him, and staying five weeks.

The rich celebrity patients from overseas are still welcome, but increasingly hospitals are seeking out the larger number of ordinary citizens from abroad. An Argentine labor union has signed a deal with the New England Medical Center in Boston to handle the more complicated medical cases of its insurees. Among the first Argentine patients were a shop clerk receiving a kidney transplant and a retired schoolteacher being treated for breast cancer, with more to follow.

Dr. Jeffrey A. Gelfand, physician-chief at the hospital, explains that the typical bill for a domestic patient is $8,000, but because the foreign patients often have more complex illnesses, the fee for them is from to $20,000 to $30,000, with much greater profit for the hospital.

The foreign medical trade is no small business. A former official at St. Luke's Episcopal Hospital in Houston estimates that 60,000 foreigners are admitted to U.S. hospitals a year, and 350,000 more for outpatient and physician treatment. The practice is growing. Johns Hopkins says that its care for foreign patients has grown twelvefold in just two years. Americans complain about the cost of hospital care here, but an Argentine cardiologist, formerly of Yale, says that many complex illnesses can be treated here more cheaply than in his country.

It May Look and Sound Like a Nurse, But . . .

Staying alive includes one large move by many hospitals that is quite detrimental to quality medicine. That is cutting down the number of registered nurses (R.N.s) and replacing them with untrained lay personnel—one of the reasons for the death of the young woman discussed at the beginning of this chapter.

The move makes economic sense. R.N.s earn from $40,000 to $50,000 on average, and hospitals can hire a "patient care technician," what used to be called "nurses' aides," for half that amount. R.N.s either have a two-year college training certificate, or a bachelor's degree in nursing science, or even postgraduate work, and are licensed by the state. On the other hand, the typical "aide," no matter what the title, generally has only six weeks training and no basic understanding of the health sciences.

To the nurses, the new movement, which is quickly replacing R.N.s with laypeople at the bedside, is not only a threat to their professional health, but to that of the sick patient as well. As costs become paramount, the number of nurses in relation to all bedside care persons is being reduced. The situation of less nurses per patient exists throughout the nation but is most extreme in California, where there are more for-profit hospitals than anywhere in the nation, and therefore, where the cost of medicine is most paramount in decision-making.

When Alta Bates Medical Center in Berkeley began what they call "patient-focused" care, they decided to cut out a good portion of the higher-paid nurses' jobs, replacing them with unlicensed "care associate" personnel. The R.N.s will do more supervisory work, but the nursing associations say their real value is alongside the patient.

"The patient should ask if the person doing the bedside care is an R.N.," says a spokesperson at the American Nurses Association. "If not, they should ask the hospital to get them an R.N. It's the best thing for their health."

The California Nurses Association, fearful of the impact of profit-making hospitals, sued the Alta Bates Medical Center for "patient deception" in that the hospital never explains the credentials of the person caring for the patient.

"Nurses have a duty to meet their regulatory obligation to make sure patients have informed consent," the attorney for their lawsuit says. "If we can't convince the courts of that, then we're going to have an entire restructuring of health services in secret."

In March 1998, the suit was settled. The HMO will now allow the nurses to help monitor the quality of care given to their patients. Northern California nurses can now appoint "quality liaison nurses" to serve as watchdogs in Kaiser hospitals. "People want some assurance that they can get the care they need when they need it. And they've always trusted the nurse at the bedside to be their advocate."

Solutions to the Hospital Crisis

The American hospital is in crisis, especially now that costs often replace quality as the ultimate criterion. Can the patient and taxpayer do anything to change the situation, stabilize the chaos, and arrive at a hospital system that is designed for the patient, and not for outside interests?

The answer is yes, and we can offer this eight-point plan as a starting place.

I. All nursing care should be provided by individuals who have no less than one year of health sciences training after high school. No one else should be permitted to take vital signs, dispense medication, and evaluate the patient's progress under doctor's orders.

II. Each hospital should tabulate and declare its infection rate to the Joint Commission on Accreditation each year, and such material should be published for all hospitals, in print, and on the Internet. Each hospital should prove that it is fully following the guidelines of the CDC or lose their Joint Commission accreditation.

III. Each state should pass legislation prohibiting the operation of for-profit hospitals in their state. For a community or public hospital to cut costs to continue operating is one thing. To cut costs to make a profit off sickness is an evil idea and should be made illegal everywhere. Those profit hospitals, some 750 now in business, should be purchased by the community, the city, or the state. Connecticut has no for-profit hospitals, a policy that should become nationwide.

IV. Every three years, every hospital should be required to conduct a survey, carried out by an independent outside organization, on the extent of iatrogenic illness and death, plus the incidence of all errors, including surgery, medical care, bedside care, and pharmaceuticals. Such information, identified according to the name of the hospital, should be disseminated by Medicare, Medicaid, HMOs, the Joint Commission, and the American Hospital Association.

V. The number of hospitals should be reduced by some fifteen percent so the financial pressure on each remaining hospital is lessened, as will be the number of empty beds.

VI. The departments of health of each state should conduct a study, at least every two years, on the success of such common operations as bypass surgery and angioplasty, as does New York State. In addition, they should publish risk-adjusted figures on breast cancer recovery and other common illnesses, along with the rates of unnecessary surgery as compiled by an independent board of surgeons.

VII. The Joint Commission should immediately publish the names of hospitals that have been refused accreditation or had it taken away from them. At present, that action is kept secret.

VIII. An ombudsman organization should be created in every state to intercede for disgruntled patients who believe their hospital bills are too high. Those organizations would be set up by the legislatures, and their decisions would have the power of law, requiring insurance companies and hospitals to obey. This is especially important since everyone acknowledges that hospital bill inflation has reached its zenith and has little to do with the patient's own care.

A lot needs to be done to make the American hospital system more stable and to *uniformly improve the quality of care.* Right now, hospitals operate in a near-anarchical way, doing much as they please, without citizen and patient overview.

This has to be changed. Hopefully, this exploration and set of recommendations will go a long way in making the American hospital what it's supposed to be—a center of healing, not horror.

Chapter III

The Epidemic of
Medical Thievery

Our Hypocritical–Not
Hippocratic–Physicians

The Medicare patient was surprised, even a touch shocked, by the doctor's bill.

He had a mild case of adult onset diabetes that he partially controlled with a few pills a day. He was used to paying $45 a visit to his internist, who had been caring for him. But he decided to seek out specialist care and went to an endocrinologist in his suburban Connecticut town.

The specialist insisted on *immediate* payment at the end of the visit. The patient could regain part of it from Medicare later on.

"But this bill of almost a hundred dollars for the visit seems too high," he told the specialist's nurse as he reached for his checkbook.

"Oh, no, Medicare approves that amount, she responded, a touch haughtily. "We just follow their guidelines."

After five visits, he totaled up the bill. It was $450, of which he was personally responsible for the fifteen percent above the Medicare-approved amount, plus twenty percent of the approved amount, or some $145. Considering that he paid Medicare monthly premiums, plus Medicare taxes of some 2.5 percent of his entire income (he was self-employed), and premiums for a Medigap policy, the out-of-pocket expense seemed excessive.

Almost a hundred dollars per simple visit, he thought to himself. At first just irritated, he finally decided on action.

He called the hot line of the Medicare fraud unit (1-800-HHS-TIPS) run by the Inspector General's Office, expecting little. To his surprise, within sixty days he received a letter from the insurance company handling Medicare in his area. They had investigated, and his suspicions were correct. Of the $450 bill, almost $200 was an overcharge. The doctor would be required to send him the refund, part of which he had to return to Medicare.

The Failed Honor System

How had the doctor, who may have been bilking his other patients as well, gotten away with the scam? Simple. Medicare is on the honor system, and apparently there is less and less honor among American physicians these days than ever before. What the doctor did, Medicare learned, was simply check off a higher-priced government code—that is, he "upcoded" the form, or "billed too high a level of care." It was as if this simple case was as complex as a sensitive diabetic being controlled by insulin treatment several times a day.

A slight shift of the pen, and violà, the doctor was becoming rich at taxpayers' expense.

Is this an isolated case?

Hardly. We must assume that most doctors are still honest, but a pernicious epidemic of dishonesty has infected the medical profession and is helping to bankrupt

Medicare, Medicaid, and the health insurance industry. It infects not just the fee-for-service physician, but the hospitals, the HMOs, the dentists who are compensated by Medicaid and private insurers, the medical equipment distributors, the testing laboratories, the home care industry, the nursing homes, and virtually everyone who calls himself a "health provider."

Everyone in the medical industry, which takes in $1 trillion year, may be involved. But at the center of the fraud, almost by legal necessity, is the prime provider, the American physician. As a special fraud counsel for the U.S. Attorney in South Florida has pointed out, it is usually a case of *cherchez le docteur*. In "all fraud cases," he says, "somewhere along the line there's a physician involved."

It is not organized crime, just an enormous cottage industry that is ingeniously and creatively ripping off America to the tune of some $100 billion dollars a year, and perhaps much more.

Other People's Money

Why are there so many crooks in what used to be a reputable profession.

The answer is "OPM"—Other People's Money. Apparently, bilking a third party like the government or an insurance fund doesn't seem to trigger the conscience of the profession as much as *directly* picking the pockets of patients they are sworn to respect and cure. It is a sick rationalization, because whether in taxes or premiums, the patients are the ones who eventually pay for the colossal industry that takes in one in every seven dollars of the Gross Domestic Product, and processes *four billion* claims a year for insurance payments.

The ease with which fraud is conducted shocks even the medical crooks.

A Philadelphia cardiologist was convicted of stealing $500,000 by making false claims to both government and private insurance systems in three states. Testifying before a U.S. Senate committee, he said he was surprised that his claims were ever paid. "The problem is that nobody is watching," he told the legislators. "The system is extremely easy to evade. The forms I sent in were absolutely outrageous. I was astounded when some of those payments were made."

Is this a case of a few bad apples in a bushel of untarnished McIntosh? Surely not. The Office of the Inspector General of the Department of Health and Human Services has recouped more than $1 billion in fines and restitutions involving only the federal health programs in the past decade.

Just the government's "overpayment" of bills submitted by providers of Medicare comes to $23 billion a year, or almost fifteen percent of all Medicare fee-for-service payments, says an audit of the aged care system. This, of course, is the proverbial icy tip. Malcolm Sparrow, a lecturer at Harvard's Kennedy School of Government, believes that just the Medicare fraud could be as large as $63 billion a year, more than a third of the total cost of the program.

In all, the estimated $100 billion a year in health care fraud is probably understated, especially since policing is lax. There are less than five hundred agents in the FBI and 250 in the government's Inspector General's Office assigned to the problem—dealing with 720,000 doctors, 190,000 dentists (many of whom collect through Medicaid), some 6,200 hospitals, and over 1,000 HMOs.

Widespread Fraud

As FBI Director Louis Freeh testified to Congress about medical thievery: "The crime problem is so big and so diverse that we are making only a small dent in addressing the fraud." June Gibbs Brown, the Inspector General at HHS, adds that the Medicare program is "inherently at high risk" for fraud.

The private sector is equally fertile ground for crooked

doctors and hospitals. According to the Health Insurance Association of America, a survey of 105 insurers turned up 43,000 new cases of suspected fraud, a rise of one-third in just two years.

The medical crooks are ingenious and getting bolder every day. The fraud schemers range from doctors to the large profit-making medical organizations, some of whom view fraud as just another income-producing stream. The General Accounting Office, the investigative arm of the U.S. Congress, reported, for example, that ABC Home Health, Inc. (later known as First American Health Care), the nation's largest home health care provider, had filed $14 million in fraudulent billings. According to the Inspector General of HHS handling the case, that included many items "solely for the personal use and enjoyment of its owners"—even a BMW for the owner's son!

Their extravagant and creative take, which resulted in convictions of mail fraud and other violations against the company and its CEO, included such goodies as:

- Utility costs and maid service for luxury beach condominiums (notice plural)
- Promotional items, including $84,341 in gourmet popcorn
- Golf course membership, green fees, and purchases at the pro shop
- Airplane and auto expenses for personal trips
- Lobbying expenses, such as ninety-eight bags of onions sent to legislators
- Alcoholic beverages on a vast scale, totaling almost $1 million

This list should be paralyzing to anyone paying his monthly premiums and exorbitant Medicare taxes, which are now linked to everyone's *full income* and not just to Social Security's $68,000 limit.

Cheaters of Quality

And just because an organization is nonprofit doesn't mean that it will ignore a chance for creative accounting that favors them and drains the near-bankrupt Medicare fund.

Nor does medical quality have a bearing on the desire to cheat. Massachusetts General Hospital, which is connected to Harvard Medical School and is one of the leading teaching hospitals in the nation, was fined $418,094 for submitting false claims to the government for work done by its physicians—a somewhat higher fine than that paid by the Boston University Medical Center.

A common scam among prestigious teaching hospitals is double-billing. The hospitals receive Medicare money for the teaching of their medical residents, as much as $100,000 a year for each postgraduate student. But they still often try to double-bill these young doctors as part of their "faculty practice." The scheme is a simple but ingenious end run that robs the Medicare fund.

The University of Pennsylvania and its faculty practice plan refunded $30 million for that unseemly practice, while Thomas Jefferson University paid $12 million to settle similar claims. In fact, some forty faculty practices at medical colleges have been investigated for that scam.

The medical schools have invented other ways to cheat Medicare. At one Boston institution, Medicare received a $177,000 reimbursement when two departments of the college—cardiology and radiology—got together to tap Uncle Sam. Since cardiologists cannot bill Medicare for interpretation of coronary angiograms, but radiologists can, the radiology department billed Medicare, then paid kickbacks to the cardiology group. Again, it was confirmation that quality and honesty don't necessarily go together.

But the larger money scams usually take place in private, for-profit medical operations. One racket-busting effort run by the Inspector General of HHS, called

"Operation Restore Trust," recently swept through five states. It came up with the criminal conviction of three dozen people, including seven doctors. The program, which still has over two hundred cases under investigation, has come away with $42 million in fines and restitution from medical thieves.

One convicted doctor in California was sentenced to eighteen months in prison for billing Medicare more than $100,000 for fictitious psychotherapy services given nursing home patients. The macabre aspect of the case was that many of the patients were, as the IG stated, "mentally incompetent and could not have benefited even if [the doctor] had been present," as he often was not.

The Brink's Heist of Medicine

Some medical crooks have high ambition, setting their sights on massive raids on the federal treasury. One California ophthalmologist pulled off the medical equivalent of the Brink's heist when he billed Medicare for the unbelievable amount of *$46 million* over a period of four years—or almost $12 million a year. According to the government, he created a "surgery mill," in which he falsified patient records to justify numerous unnecessary cataract and eyelid operations. In addition to this wholesale theft, he put his patients through unneeded pain and worry.

Another doctor, this one in New York, didn't bother with unnecessary medical care. He just billed Medicaid for $13 million over a period of eighteen months. Since caring for that many patients in such a short time is physically impossible, the greedy physician managed it by eliminating one vital step in the process. He didn't bother to see the patients at all. He merely marked on their medical records that he had treated them, then billed Medicaid for the nonvisits.

The operating law in prosecuting medical fraud is the False Claims Act. First passed during the Civil War, it rewarded whistle-blowers when they reported shoddy or nonexistent work by wartime profiteers. The award was a piece of the money recovered when the thieves were caught.

This obscure piece of legislation has now been reborn. It was amended in 1986, and fines of $10,000 and triple damages for *each* false claim were levied. This has resulted in a tenfold increase in fraud reporting just since 1992. The patient can not only gain the satisfaction of reporting a crooked doctor, but take home a reward of up to 25 percent of the money recovered from sizable scams.

Extra Blood Tests

In the case of Damon Clinical Laboratories, once the largest medical laboratory in America (since purchased by Corning, Inc. and spun off as Quest Diagnostics), medical immorality reached a new low. The laboratory fooled physicians by making expensive additional tests of serum iron and putting them in with the routine blood screening even though the doctors had never ordered the extra tests.

An HHS investigator who worked on the case explains that an automated blood sampler checks nineteen items at once for only $10. But just a single "serum ferriten" test—the type fraudulently made by Damon—costs more than all the others combined. The whistle-blowers were rewarded with grants of up to $9 million, and the lab pled guilty to criminal charges and paid $119 million in fines, penalties and recovered monies, three times what it bilked from federal health programs. In 1998, four top executives of Damon were indicted for criminal fraud and have pleaded not guilty. The case highlights the devilish indecency now invading the health care business.

Some of this is, paradoxically, legal. It falls into the category of extraordinary waste. Medicare pays—says the Office of the Inspector General—"nearly twice as much as physicians for the same tests." Why? It turns out that labs offer groups of tests to doctors at greatly reduced prices while Medicare usually pays the fee schedule rates for individual tests. (Medicare now says it is *trying* to reduce the waste.)

Lab scams are among the most outrageous cases of medical mischief. The Laboratory Corporation of America agreed to pay $182 million to settle civil charges that one of its predecessor companies submitted false claims to both federal and state health programs. That predecessor, Allied Clinical Laboratories, admitted to a criminal count of fraudulent billing of Medicare by its San Diego laboratory. Not only did they pay $5 million in fines, but they have been banned from ever dealing with Medicare or Medicaid, the real cake-and-caviar of the lab industry.

In one case, patients billed were not only not tested, but were not really available. A billing clerk in Florida, wife of the firm's president, submitted 717 claims for 416 patients, and received $330,000 in payment from Medicare. The problem was that many of the "patients" were dead. In fact, one of the supposedly "referring" doctors had passed away two years before.

In all, the government has recovered more than $600 million from its investigation of diagnostic labs, whose work, in most cases, is fully covered by the government at no extra cost to Medicaid and Medicare patients.

Convoluted Medicare Codes

But for every medical scammer that is caught, another half dozen seem to appear. They are all helped by Medicare rules, which are as convoluted and confusing as the IRS code. The Medicare rule book, with thirty years of clarifications and interpretations, runs to 45,000 pages! Even the manuals of local insurance carriers alone weigh in at two thousand pages. Little wonder it brings out the creative streak in health providers.

The code is unwieldy and subject to manipulation, generally in favor of the doctor or hospital, and against the patient (who directly pays part of the bill) and the government, where the taxpayer eventually pays all of it.

Alice C. Gosfield, a Philadelphia attorney who is an expert on health care, explains the procedure a doctor goes through to get paid. It involves 10,000 CPT (Current Procedural Terminology) codes, which can be combined into more than 99,000 permutations. If the doctor wants to take in more cash than he (or increasingly, she) should, he can easily manipulate the system—one that seems designed to encourage crooks. If a patient comes in with a headache, Ms. Gosfield explains, the doctor may:

- Charge Medicare for a procedure that didn't take place
- Bill them for more time than was actually spent with the patient
- "Upcode" the procedure to get more money for his care, as the endocrinologist did, by checking off a more complex, more expensive treatment than the one actually performed
- "Unbundle," or separate, each procedure of the patient visit, or parts of a lab test, and bill them separately with separate codes, bringing in more money than by merely checking off a single explanatory code.

The Upcoding Scam

"Upcoding" is the easiest way to defraud the insurer, government or private. In the case of the giant Empire Blue Cross/Blue Shield in New York, investigators found many cases of upcoding.

The Empire billing code for an upper respiratory infection, for example, is 465.9, a code that calls for about a $125 fee for the doctor. But by simply filling in the code 490.2, which is for a bronchial problem, the doctor can collect an additional fifty dollars from the insurer. Going to code 99245, which represents a consultation for a severe problem, the payment can jump to $300 or more.

"Doctors can put down any variety of codes within a

certain range, and unless we catch them in a pattern, which is very hard since there are more than seven thousand codes, they're going to get away with it," Empire's antifraud head, Lou Parisi, former chief of the state's Insurance Fraud Division, has pointed out.

The possibilities of fraud under the "honor" system are endless. This is especially true since there are few routine, random spot checks of doctors, as the IRS does with its regular audits of 2 million taxpayers a year.

One Pennsylvania ob/gyn specialist had to pay back $98,000 to Medicare and a private insurer for twisting the truth. He billed Medicare for Pap smears that he never performed, then toyed with the "codes" by marking routine office visits with pregnant women as "emergencies." He also billed for hospital services that had already been paid to the hospital.

On Long Island, a physician practiced minor cosmetic surgery by injecting patients with collagen to smooth out wrinkles and puff up deflated lips. He knew that the procedures were not covered by either Medicare or private insurers. To collect, he claimed that he had performed other medical procedures, including bronchoscopy and laryngoscopies.

When the private insurance company became suspicious, they contacted the FBI. The tragic aspect of the case is that the physician had been an army surgeon in Vietnam, decorated for bravery under fire. His honor, however, seemed to fail him when he started practicing medicine.

A Psychiatric Crook

A Boston area psychiatrist did more than toy with the codes. His scheme to defraud Medicare, Medicard, and a private insurer only confirmed the public stereotype that certain members of his specialty are less than stable. He filed hundreds of false claims, some for more therapy sessions than he actually conducted, and others for patients he never saw.

But the billing fiasco was only the beginning of his mad escapade. Once he became aware of the investigation, he called the patients involved and desperately sought to get them to lie for him. Then he extended his web of deceit by threatening a potential witness. If she cooperated with the government, he would—he warned—go public with the psychiatric medical records of a member of her family. Fortunately, the witness refused to be intimidated.

As the case went to court as a civil trial for Medicare fraud and a criminal one for Medicaid, the psychiatrist grasped for his last option. He pled insanity, claiming he suffered from a psychotic delusion that caused him to overbill insurers.

One overbiller didn't bother with such mundane procedures as psychotherapy. A heart surgeon in Colorado stretched his imagination far enough to invent heart bypass operations he never performed!

Sometimes physician chicanery is the result of doctors entering the deep waters of entrepreneurship, where there is always the danger of conflict of interest between patient care and making a buck—too often a quick, dishonest buck.

One Illinois physician was sentenced to two years in jail for using fraud in trying to rescue a failing multimillion-dollar diagnostic clinic he had built. When he couldn't get enough referrals from doctors to make it pay, he billed every patient who visited the clinic between $4,000 and $6,000 in unnecessary tests. To make matters worse, he tried to justify the billings by entering "false symptoms" in the patients' records. The trial lasted five months, the longest in the southern Illinois district.

Home Care Fraud

Fraud is rampant in all areas of medicine, but its increasing most rapidly in the burgeoning business of home health care. This service, covered by both Medicare and Medicaid, is designed for the homebound aged and seriously ill returning from the hospital. To receive home health care, a Medicare patient must be homebound and under the care of a doctor, who certifies his case and outlines treatment.

The system has zoomed to new heights in recent years, with 25,000 firms entering the business. In 1990 it cost Medicare $3.3 billion, but by 1994 that had risen to $12 billion, and is estimated today at almost $20 billion a year. The number of patients has grown simultaneously, from 1.9 to 5 million.

Because Washington thought home care would be cheaper than longer hospital stays, it set up a system that encourages fraud. Medicare agreed to *reimburse home care providers in full for all their costs.* With the growth of the program has come some frauds that rival the best (or worst) television dramas, as we have already seen in the bold illegal scheme of ABC Home Health, Inc.

In Dade County, Florida, five doctors have been charged with fraud in a massive home health care swindle, part of a 102-count indictment being prosecuted by the U.S. Attorney for South Florida. The scheme, which involved officials of Mederi of Dade County, a home health agency, was extra bold. Seven defendants pled guilty; twelve including the corporation, are going to trial.

In return for sizable kickbacks, physicians allegedly signed home health certifications and plans of treatment for patients they had never seen. According to Wilfredo Fernandez, special counsel for the U. S. Attorney, the doctors were part of a conspiracy to bilk $15 million from Medicare: "In literally thousands of claims, to date we have not found one person who received services in the cases covered in the indictments."

Another home health fraud involved a Georgia-based firm. The government has accused them of perpetrating a "conspiracy to defraud the Medicare program of millions of dollars through the submission of fraudulent cost reports." The company has allegedly sought reimbursement for political contributions, pleasure trips, and payments to "related" companies actually owned and controlled by officers of the firm. In effect, they were pilfering the taxpayer on behalf of several companies all at the same time.

Lure of Government Cash

Like the Mafia and Hollywood, the big monies involved in Medicare and Medicaid—over $400 billion a year—attract the unsavory. Once the facts of the fraud are unraveled, they often seem bizarre, as if the medical crooks never expected to be checked, which unfortunately is often the case.

St. Johns Home Health Agency was one of those that did happen to be checked. The Inspector General found that fully *three-fourths* of their claims did not meet Medicare guidelines, including several that smack of chicanery:

- 21.5 percent of the claims were for visits *never made*
- 29 percent were to individuals who were not homebound, as required
- 23.5 percent were for visits doctors said were not authorized by them

Even the temporary help giant, the Olsten Corporation, has become involved in a federal investigation. Stimulated by government largesse, they entered the home health business and have since acquired or opened five hundred such agencies nationwide, in addition to managing four hundred more for others. In July 1997, FBI agents walked into twenty-two Florida offices that Olsten managed for the troubled Columbia/HCA chain and took out hundreds of documents and diskettes. As of now, the Justice Department is trying to learn if Olsten has been overbilling the taxpayer.

One of the fastest growing aspects of home health care is "infusion therapy," a method of taking intravenous treatments at home. Covered by Medicare, it now runs some $5 billion a year. Says the Inspector General's Office: "We believe that kickbacks in the form of case management fees or fees for service are used as incentives for physicians to refer patients to a particular company. Payment averages $150 per week per patient. Doctors have made $10,000 per month in kickbacks."

In one case, the government suspected that a home health care firm gave gifts to the head of hematology at the University of New Mexico Hospital, ostensibly to encourage him to make referrals. Days after his office was searched by the FBI, he killed himself.

Kickback scams are omnipresent in medicine. Dishonest and ingenious doctors can take in sums much greater than $100,000 a year. In one case involving Caremark International, a Minneapolis-based home care company, a federal grand jury indicted them for paying astronomical kickbacks to one physician. How much? Caremark pleaded guilty to mail fraud and paid a fine of $161 million. Suprisingly, the doctor was convicted but that conviction was overturned on appeal; the charges against the executives were dismissed entirely.

After an investigation of Caremark by the FBI, the HHS Inspector General, and the Minnesota Health Care Fraud Task Force, several physicians and executives were charged with an elaborate plot. The charge was based on a law that bars renumeration for referrals. According to the government, the company paid the doctor, a pediatric endocrinologist, $1.1 million in kickbacks to induce him to prescribe a human growth hormone, Protropin, which was distributed to doctors exclusively by Caremark. The doctor was one of the nation's largest prescribers of the drug.

Nursing Home Cheats

Nursing homes, like home health care, are another growing arena for taxpayer-paid medicine. Today, over 1 million beneficiaries—the aged and those leaving hospitals who need skilled nursing care—are covered by Medicare Part A, the hospitalization segment. Medicare Part B covers the cost of doctors, lab work, ambulance, and medical supplies for 2 million patients in nursing homes. Medicaid covers nursing home care for the poor over the age of twenty-one, and now numbers some 3 million patients at a cost of some $35 billion a year, paid by both the states and Washington. (And all by taxpayers.)

Overall, the annual *public* nursing care bill for America is well past $50 billion a year. A large, if unknown, portion of this is stolen by fraudulent firms and physicians.

One of the most profitable scams involves medical equipment and supplies, especially those purchased by nursing homes with Medicare or Medicaid funds. Some equipment sellers, referred to as DME (Durable Medical Equipment) firms, seem to be among the boldest of medical thiefs. In one recent four-year period, there were 131 successful criminal prosecutions of medical suppliers or their employees. Little wonder, since Medicare does almost no background checks, making the federal treasury a fertile source for scam artists. In one case an owner had even been convicted of murder.

An Illinois entrepreneur was sentenced to five months in jail and five months home confinement for defrauding Medicare by obtaining the Social Security numbers of nursing home patients. He then forged doctors' names on claim forms for wheelchairs and beds he never delivered.

An ingenious scam was to soak the government by seeking payment for "orthotic body jackets," customized rigid devices meant to hold patients with muscular and spinal conditions immobile in order to reduce their pain.

Payment for these jackets went from $217,000 in 1990 to $18 million just two years later. How was that possible? Investigators learned that most of it was fraudulent—that ninety-five percent of the payments were actually for devices better described as "seat cushions" than as rigid jackets.

That was the core of a racket perpetrated by a Texas firm whose three principals were convicted for having bought seat pads manufactured in Mexico for fifty dollars each, then billing Medicare $1,200 for each as "body jackets." The owner of a nursing home who participated in the Texas firm's gimmick was bribed with a free $500,000 life insurance policy.

Abusing the Incontinent

Supplies for the incontinent (mainly aged), who can no longer control their body's bowels or bladder, are heavily loaded with fraud as well. Medicare covers long-term or indefinite incontinence, including accessories such as drainage bags, irrigation syringes, and sterile saline solutions. But for some reason, probably cost, it does *not* include absorbent undergarments like those peddled on television by World War II actress June Allyson.

The incontinent have proven a gold mine for *fraudmeisters*. From an $88-million cost of such supplies in 1990, it suddenly rose to $230 million in 1993, and even more today. Oddly, the number of incontinent patients actually fell during that same period.

One favorite scam was the marketing of "incontinence kits" to nursing homes. The potential for profit was enormous. In a report to the House Subcommittee on Health, the Deputy Inspector General reported that "the cost of supplies contained in an incontinence kit is typically four dollars.

"These items are fragmented [unbundled] and upcoded for billing purposes, causing Medicare to be billed about twenty dollars for each kit," he explained. "Providers usually ship and bill at the rate of three kits per day per beneficiary, which is the maximum that Medicare will reimburse. At ninety kits per month, the cost to Medicare Part B is $1,800 per month, per patient. It is not surprising that this has turned into a $200-million business."

How come, and how widespread is the practice? The answer is shocking.

"We believe that questionable billing practices may account for almost half of Medicare allowances for incontinent supplies," the Inspector General says. She adds that "unscrupulous suppliers engage in questionable marketing practices," including falsely advising nursing homes that *they* could decide on the amount of these supplies that Medicare would pay for.

Of the $6 billion spent on medical supplies each year, at least a third overall, perhaps more, goes into the coffers of fraudulent operators.

Medical Equipment Scams

The aged are the most common victims of the medical equipment scammers, who usually need the help of unsavory doctors to pull off their illegal schemes. Some accomplish this by paying unethical physicians to sign "Certificates of Medical Necessity" (CMT), the indispensable open sesame to the racket. In other cases they just forge the doctor's name.

Two brothers in New York were convicted of an ingenious scheme that involved throwing "health fairs," where senior citizens were coaxed to divulge their Medicare numbers. The brothers gave these numbers, along with forged CMTs, to two medical equipment companies authorized by Medicare. The companies then billed Medicare $750,000 for equipment, much of which was never supplied. The brothers received "commissions," actually thinly disguised kickbacks.

In another medical equipment fraud case in New York, physicians were actively involved in the scam, a massive one involving $13 million in payments from Medicare. The sales people solicited the names and numbers of naive Medicare patients. The doctors signed the fake CMTs, for which they received kickbacks. The company then filed the multimillion-dollar claims for equipment never supplied.

Other medical equipment frauds include the following cornucopia of inventive schemes:

The owner of one firm pled guilty to a conspiracy to defraud Medicare. The scheme, called "carrier shopping," billed for items sold from California to Florida, after the perpetrators determined in which states Medicare paid the highest reimbursements. Using shell offices or mail drops, they pretended to do business in those states. The owners and top management were arrested and indicted.

Some DME scammers work by phone. In Pennsylvania they solicited Medicare beneficiaries by telephone at home, then sold them bed pads designed to protect those suspectible to sores. But many of the patients were fully ambulatory and didn't need, nor did they use, the pads. The patients' records had been altered in several cases to justify the sales and entries made in other than the doctors' handwriting. The owner was sentenced to jail.

One Ohio firm aggressively telemarketed motorized wheelchairs, but provided electric scooters instead. They billed Medicare for the price of the wheelchair—$5,000— instead of the $2,000 for the scooters.

The latest fraud perpetrated against the aged is the *hospice racket*. As life is extended, more seniors struggle on longer before death. The legitimate answer to that problem are hospices, hospital-like settings for the terminally ill that will allow them to die in greater dignity. The result is that the hospice program is the fastest-growing aspect of the federal Medicare program, coverage that began in 1984.

But as the government and insurers become the primary payers of care, unscrupulous providers have entered the field to seek maximum, often illegal, profits. *This scam relies on enrolling patients who are not terminally ill* in hospices, siphoning them off from the nursing homes. In May 1998, federal prosecutors charged one hospice in Chicago of doing just that. Allegedly, the owner paid nursing homes for each new hospice patient, and gave doctors a monthly stipend (sometimes as little as $89) for falsely certifying that patients were terminally ill—allegedly without ever examining them.

The cost of just this one scam, according to the prosecutors, was $28.5 million! Ostensibly, the hospice population is so padded that almost one in three patients is not terminally ill and therefore not eligible. In addition, the government claims that many of the patients received substandard care and that their benefits ran out *before* they ever became terminally ill.

The question of enforcement in this and other such cases is becoming increasingly difficult. In Illinois, where the alleged hospice fraud took place, the state employs a total of twenty-nine nurses to enforce regulations at 100 hospices, 200 hospitals, 465 nursing homes, 100 dialysis centers, 150 rural health clinics, 100 ambulatory care centers, and several thousand clinical labs.

Medicare "Excludes" Doctors

Medicare does not always prosecute cases in court, but may instead punish the offenders through "exclusion." In these cases, Medicare decides—under Sections 1128(b) (6) and 1156 of the Social Security Act—that a health provider should be cut out of the system. After that they may no longer bill Medicare, even if the patient wants them to. The reasons for "exclusion," the Inspector General says, may not only be fraud, but can include blatant failure of quality care (See Chapter IV).

This was the case of a California oncologist (cancer specialist) accused of "rendering 3,900 excessive, substandard, unnecessary, and potentially risky services to seven Medicare beneficiaries over a six-year time period." He was "excluded" from collecting from Medicare for a ten-year period. Later on, because of his treatment of six Medicare patients with ten hospital admissions, he again came to the attention of federal investigators.

According to the Inspector General, the cancer specialist's newest violations included "inappropriate blood transfusion, inappropriate treatment for sepsis, and failure to detect the development of a decubitus ulcer while the patient was under medical care during a prolonged hospitalization." The physician was "excluded" from collecting from Medicare for another ten years.

Other "exclusions" cover the full spectrum.

- In a transportation scam in Louisiana, owners of the cars carrying patients to medical providers were convicted of a scheme that defrauded Medicaid of $2 million by billing the government for miles that were not actually traveled.
- Two officers of a medical equipment company were excluded from Medicare after setting up a scheme to rip off the government by providing "liquid nutritional supplements" to the aged. They had physicians sign a "Certificate of Medical Necessity" in each case, even though the doctors had never examined the patients.

Each year, Medicare "excludes" some 1,500 health providers from receiving payments, and provides the public with both a printed list and diskettes. It also enters the information on IGnet, an Internet resource from sixty federal Inspector General Offices. The list is cumulative, updated monthly, and is available at: http:www.sbaonline.sba.gov/ignet/internal/hhs/invlist/html (Of course, leave it to the government to create one of the longest Internet addresses imaginable.)

Internecine Professional Feuds

Fraud investigations have also brought to the surface feuds within the medical profession that have been kept from the public. One of these is the fight between anesthesiologists (medical doctor specialists) and nurse anesthetists, who do much of the work for the doctors but are paid considerably less.

In a *$1-billion* Medicare fraud lawsuit, nurse anesthetists in Minnesota claim that the physicians billed the government for personally performing these services even "though they were never present in the operating room with the patient and the nurse anesthetist for the entire anesthesia time as required by Medicare."

Was this just an occasional laxity or oversight—which patients can't usually observe because they're asleep? Or is it a routine doctor scam? The nurses say it is a regular ripoff that has taken place in 100,000 instances just in that state over a period of six years. In an eighty-eight-page complaint under the Federal False Claims Act, the nurses are suing sixty-five defendants, including physicians and some of the major hospitals in the state.

In a touch of whimsy, the nurses made public some of the excuses offered by the anesthesiologists for not being in the operating room trenches with them:

- They were providing services for other patients at the time they were billing Medicare for anesthesia work in the operating room
- They were sleeping
- They were reading
- Attending to personal business on the phone
- Watching *Star Trek*
- Watching Minnesota Viking football games
- Leaving the hospital

Deception in Our Hospitals

Medical racketeering has spread across the entire health care field, turning American hospitals as well into centers of deception, obfuscation, and fraud.

Hospitals are hard-pressed to stay alive. With excessive expansion, beginning with the Hill-Burton Act of the 1950s, with almost forty percent empty beds coupled with increased competition for patients and lower payments from HMOs and Medicare, hospital honesty has almost disappeared.

Federal investigators have found that of the nation's 6,200 hospitals, some 4,600 have submitted "improper" bills for outpatient services, for instance, helping to deplete Medicare's already scarce funds. The scam is simple. Medicare is billed twice for hospital nonphysician *outpatient* work—once separately, and the second time as part of the *inpatient* invoice. It is a lucrative area because in order to cut down hospitalizations, Medicare is much more generous with outpatient than with inpatient hospital work. In fact, they cover all the hospital costs—plus—rather than grant them a fee.

By the fall of 1996, 925 hospitals had confessed to this practice and promised to reform. The investigation continues, and Medicare expects to pick up $110 million in restitution and fines, probably only a small percentage of what has already been skimmed.

Double-billing by hospitals, in some form, is a common method of taking in more Medicare and Medicaid funds than they're entitled to. Without admitting that they broke any laws, four hospitals—two in Pennsylvania and two in South Dakota—returned money to the U.S. Treasury. Their shenanigan? They double-billed Medicare for laboratory tests when payment for them had already been included in their regular hospital charges.

Another hospital, this one in Colorado, agreed to reimburse the government because it had also double-billed. In this case, they charged both Medicare and the Veterans Administration for the same services!

They Call It "Revenue Enhancement"

One new technique of money-starved, patient-poor hospitals, which sounds legitimate, can spill over into outright fraud. Increasingly, hospitals are using skilled consultants to create "revenue enhancement" techniques. By hitting Medicare and Medicaid as hard as legally possible, they sometimes go over the edge, confusing "enhancement" with chicanery.

Two hospitals in Pennsylvania, the Geisinger Wyoming Valley Medical Center in Wilkes-Barre and the Warren General Hospital in Warren, were among those that tried too hard. After hiring a consultant to increase their revenue, they ended up with charges from Medicare and had to reimburse the government $424,000 and $145,000 respectively.

A Kansas medical center agreed to pay $1.2 million to settle false claims stemming from an ingenious kickback scheme. It was pulled off by a medical group composed of five hospitals located in Kansas and Missouri, which provided on-site care to nursing home patients. It was a successful medical practice, except the doctors involved paid an illegal kickback fee to the medical center for referring patients to the group. That ended up costing Medicare $500,000 in overpayments, for which the hospitals had to pay back an amount more than double their take.

The extent of hospital fraud, which is blatant, can be gauged by a report from the U.S. Attorney's Office in Massachusetts, which revealed that eighty-three hospitals in that state alone had filed false Medicare claims. Nationwide, settlements have been made with over a thousand hospitals to date, with more to come.

Why? Because the overexpanded hospital system is finding it hard to attract patients despite enormous and highly creative advertising campaigns. Unable to stay alive legitimately, they are turning to everything from overbilling to outright fraud to keep themselves in business. The obvious victim is health insurance, especially the inefficient federal government programs.

One of the largest alleged hospital fraud cases involves Columbia/HCA Healthcare Corporation, a $20-billion-a-year conglomerate that controls over three hundred hospitals and numerous HMOs and home health care companies. Not only is it the largest health care company in America, but its revenue rivals the total medical costs of some smaller *nations*.

Columbia is a for-profit institution, surely the fastest-growing and most controversial part of the American hospital system.

Raid on Columbia/HCA

Agents of the FBI, the Department of Defense Criminal Investigation Service, the Department of Health and Human Services, and the U.S. .Attorney's Office raided the company's offices in El Paso, Texas, in March 1997—seeking confirmation of their suspicions. One was that the health giant had overbilled the government and required doctors affiliated with them to send blood and other samples to labs in which the physicians had ownership brokered by Columbia/HCA.

By July 1997, agents had seized documents from more than thirty-five Columbia hospitals and their offices in seven states, seeking proof of suspected fraud. Richard Scott, the firm's CEO, resigned, replaced by Thomas Frist, Jr., the vice-chairman, whose family had founded the forerunner Hospital Corporation of America in the 1960s.

On July 31, 1997, three mid-level executives of the hospital conglomerate—who had been busily buying up both for-profit and voluntary community hospitals over the years—were indicted for a "conspiracy" to inflate the amount of money Columbia was to be reimbursed by both Medicare and Champus, the military health insurance plan. A fourth executive was later charged. All have denied the charges.

Part of the indictment involves Columbia's activity in their Fawcett Memorial Hospital in Port Charlotte, Florida, which Columbia bought in 1992. The government now charges that the three indicted men allegedly developed a scheme to have Medicare and Champus totally reimburse the hospital for its debt load, a gimmick that ostensibly cost the taxpayers $1.75 million.

The Columbia case, which is still being probed by the FBI, has yet to be played out in full. Eventually it may cast doubt on the whole question of for-profit hospitals being in the business of making money on sickness, and adding their profits to the already stretched medical care budget.

Private insurers are looking at Columbia as well, trying to learn if they too were bilked by the one-time Wall Street darling. "Columbia's troubles will not be over even if there is a settlement with the government," says Alison Duncan, a Washington attorney whose firm specializes in health care fraud. Working for some of the largest private insurers, her firm is delving into possible bilking at Columbia, which gets sixty percent of its revenue from private insurers.

The Insurers' Conflicts of Interest

This is a bit of a precedent since private health insurance companies have previously put their heads in the sand when it came to hospitals. They had an in-built conflict of interest as they strove (and strive) to become partners in the hospital business.

"Many insurers were reluctant to look for fraud and abuse because they were busy setting up their managed care network and needed the providers," the president of New York's Empire Blue Cross/Blue Shield has stated. Now, that is changing, but only out of necessity.

The Columbia case continues, with new suspicions leaking out regularly. The latest revelation involves soaking Uncle Sam by kiting the true figures. In one case involving Southwest Regional Medical Center in Fort Myers, Florida—which became part of the giant Columbia chain—officials allegedly padded their real estate taxes by $68,000, getting reimbursement for the fiction from the government.

Allegedly, they set aside the padded amount, ready to pay it back if caught. They waited a couple of years until they were audited. If the Inspector General's people failed to catch it, then the $68,000 was moved into the profit column, enhancing their Wall Street numbers, which was the core of the for-profit medical racket to begin with. At its peak in the spring of 1997, the stock sold for $86 a share, but has since dropped to the low twenties. Talk is that the government investigators will not end the case until they find *billions* in misappropriated taxpayer money.

While the government, including the FBI, was probing, the *New York Times* set out on its own investigation, turning up the following allegations:

1. Outside accountants, including the esteemed KPMG Peat Marwick, were allegedly aware that Columbia was cheating the government, and in some situations actually helped advance the deception.
2. Supervisors told employees to hide telltale documents. At one Arkansas hospital owned by Columbia, the records were stamped "CONFIDENTIAL: Do not discuss or release to Medicare auditors."
3. Expenses were inflated so they could get higher compensation from Medicare and Medicaid.
4. Columbia had much larger administrative costs than either voluntary or even other stockholder-owned hospitals. Columbia is suspected of hiding this by shifting those costs to their home care companies, where administration took about half (49.55 percent) of their total spending!

Washington Encourages Fraud

Columbia has apparently played fast and furious with government money, but we should not excuse Washington, which typically has set up a system that encourages fraud. These hospitals pose as free enterprise institutions and get all the benefits of Wall Street–type largesse, including a $10-million severance package for its ex-chief, Richard Scott, who resigned when the probe made headlines.

But, in typical federal manner, all the for-profit hospitals are subsidized with taxpayer money, just as our farmers were for years. All expenses related to patient care are reimbursed by the government.

This is an idiotic concept in a supposed capitalist enterprise, and clever hospital administrators take advantage of the government's naiveté. "Cost-reporting" is an easy opportunity for hospitals to cheat. If they are caught, all they risk is having to pay back the money, creating a unique interest-free loan.

"It's a bizarre world," says James Plonsey, a cost-reporting specialist. "There is an incentive to abuse the system, and wait for Medicare to catch you. And there has been no penalty for doing it."

This permissiveness can result in a funny kind of capitalism, one operated at the taxpayers' expense. A favorite trick of privately owned hospitals has been to "recapture" money from the government. This happens when there is a takeover of another hospital, which was Columbia's main method of growth. Columbia's acquisition of a Miami Beach hospital, for instance, was so structured that they didn't pay a cent for the hospital, yet received $24.7 million of "recaptured" money from Washington.

An investigation by Medicare revealed that the practice was widespread. In one recent year, hospitals took in $150 million in government funds using the technique. Little wonder Medicare is constantly short of cash.

Scamming the Mentally Ill

In the world of make-a-buck hospitals, psychiatric institutions often emerge as among the greatest fraud operators. Because of the effectiveness of modern psychochemicals, which allows the mentally ill to be ambulatory, those hospitals have had a difficult time getting enough inpatients. Equally important, many of them have schemed to keep their patients in the hospital long enough to satisfy their bottom line.

In one classic case, investigators cracked down and recovered a fortune from National Medical Enterprises, Inc., the parent company of a chain of eighty-two psychiatric hospitals that had been operating in twenty-six states under the name Psychiatric Institutes of America. They were successfully charged with fraud, including paying large kickbacks to doctors for recommending patients and *for not permitting patients to leave the hospitals until their insurance ran out.*

A former company executive who oversaw their operations in Texas, told a federal judge in Dallas that in a five-year period, the company paid as much as $40 million in kickbacks to doctors, therapists, and even social workers who steered patients to their hospitals. Meetings were held on a monthly basis to conspire to pay kickbacks and to disguise them as operating costs in their reports to Medicare.

As a result of the investigation, National Medical Enterprises offered a guilty plea agreement and paid the largest penalty and reimbursement in history—$33 million in criminal fines; $324.2 million in damages, restitution, and penalties; $16.3 million to several states for Medicaid claims; and $2.5 million for the National Institutes of Mental Health; for a total of $379 million.

In addition, a consortium of thirteen private insurers sued NME and collected some $200 million that had allegedly been fraudulently taken from them. Now known as Tenet Healthcare Corp., which bought out NME, the psychiatric hospital group has also agreed to pay $100 million more to settle 680 malpractice claims by patients hospitalized in its former operations in Texas.

Some seven hundred psychiatric hospitals participate in the Medicare program, and the Inspector General's Office has several investigations going on at any one time. In one recent scheme, some hospitals were illegally paying psychiatrists up to $2,000 for each patient referral, then tried to pass the cost off to Medicare. Some of the kickback money was supposedly for the writing of clinical patient manuals, which were never written.

The "Thirty-Minute" Psychiatric Hour

Psychiatry is an easy opportunity for fraud because the therapy sessions are usually time-based, much like the practice of some lawyers who bill by the classic "thirty-minute hour." One forty-eight-bed psychiatric hospital for children and adolescents from Nebraska and Tennessee hustled the Medicaid program by inflating the time spent with patients—adding an extra hour here and there. The result was that they had to return $554,700 to Medicaid.

Some greedy psychiatrists stretch the time constraints beyond reason. A Nevada psychiatrist so inflated the psychotherapy time he spent with Medicaid patients that he had to reimburse the state $300,000. He might have gotten away with it, but he made one mistake. He claimed that he spent more than twenty-four hours a day counseling his patients.

Hospital and other medical fraud is being increasingly uncovered (though only a small portion of the whole) because some people are either public-spirited or anxious to make a buck, or both. The result has been the emergence of whistle-blowers under a federal fraud tip-and-reward system set up by the Inspector General's Office.

Become a Whistle-Blower

Medicare and Medicaid patients who believe that they and the government are being taken advantage of by doctors or hospitals can call the general whistle-blower number (1-800-HHS-TIPS) and receive a reward if their lead uncovers fraud on any substantial scale.

The typical patient will just receive some money back from the doctor. But *if* investigators determine that what happened to them is endemic, penalties levied against the doctor could be large enough to trigger a substantial reward.

Most whistle-blowers are "insiders" who know what's actually going on. In the Damon Labs scam, the main whistle-blower received $9 million, the record to date. But others have received lesser amounts and a number of cases are still being processed.

Medicare fraud is handled by the federal government,

but a whole world of fraud in the Medicaid program is generally investigated by the states themselves. The Medicaid program for the poor, which now costs $200 billion a year (half paid by states) has been the fastest-growing segment of health care, mainly because it provides cradle-to-grave coverage. Unlike Medicare, it includes virtually free prescription drugs and even dental care, whose bills can reach into the thousands.

There are less patients in Medicaid than in Medicare (thirty million vs. thirty-eight million) and most of the recipients are well children instead of the chronically ill aged. Yet the costs for the two programs run about the same $200 billion each—one indication of the enormous fraud involved in Medicaid.

State Crackdown on Medicaid Fraud

The states are trying to fight widespread medical racketeering through their Medicaid Fraud Control Units, a federally funded state program operating in forty-seven states. In the nineteen years since it was founded, there have been over seven thousand convictions of medical fraud operators, which, unfortunately, represents only a small segment of the rip-off artists.

Started because of the nursing home fraud, it has now branched out to cover the whole Medicaid industry. The first crackdown came in the early 1980s when the market price of silver reached its height of fifty dollars an ounce. Immediately, X-ray photographic film became a hot item on the black market. Hospital technicians began selling the X-ray films (including actual diagnostic plates of ill patients!) to reprocessing firms, which extracted the silver.

This was no petty thievery. In some cases the fraud income came to $10,000 a month per hospital. When silver prices finally broke, the medical thieves abandoned their scam.

Foreign National Cheaters

In the mid 1980s the Medicaid frauds expanded into numerous fields, including the selling of orthopedic shoes, even acupuncture services. Some of the criminal activity was carried out by foreign nationals, who preyed on the loosely policed system.

"Within this latter group," according to a report from the National Association of Medicaid Fraud Control Units in Washington, "many maintained close contact with their native countries, made frequent trips abroad, and had no meaningful ties, other than financial, to the United States. . . . They moved from pharmacies and clinics to orthopedic shoe vendors and podiatrists, and later in the decade to sonograms and drug diversion. They became more ruthless and bold . . . because of their easy ability to flee the United States to their homeland enriched with thousands, even millions, of taxpayer dollars."

One Pakistani doctor who had practiced in the United States was apprehended at Kennedy Airport on his return from Switzerland, where he had deposited hundreds of thousands of dollars stolen from Medicaid. He had been suspended from Medicaid for unacceptable methods but continued practicing, looting the federal treasury of $1.4 million. On his arrest, authorities found he had operated under two different names and carried both U.S. and Pakistani passports.

In Southern California, investigators learned that recent immigrants from southeast Asia were being coached on how to fake psychological disability and receive payments from Medi-Cal, the state version of Medicaid. Translators and transporters, working with neighborhood medical clinics, doctors, and attorneys, kept the scheme moving. In some cases, immigrant Medicaid patients sold their "stickers" to the clinic owners, doctor, or driver so they could write their own Medicaid ticket for services.

But most of the medical fraud in America does not involve foreigners. In the main, it is expertly handled by domestic medical crooks. In New York, a physician ran an ingenious Medicaid scam. He purchased three medical test labs, then hired scouts to go out into the poor neighborhoods to offer people ten dollars for each vial of their own blood. The "scouts" were told to get as many vials as possible. Then, using the patients' Medicaid numbers, the doctor performed numerous lab tests on each "street blood" sample, charging the government as much as $2,000 per.

The Drugstore Racket

One favorite scam is for pharmacists to bill Medicaid for brand name drugs, but instead provide the Medicaid patient with much cheaper generic pharmaceuticals. Ingenious crooks have developed an even more lucrative "drugstore" racket. That scam—which Douglas Kennedy, son of the late Robert Kennedy, helped expose when on the staff of the *New York Post*—involves the prescribing, buying, then reselling of the very same drugs, a fraud that requires the connivance of several people in the health care field.

The racket operates in stages, as follows:

1. Medicaid patients visit several doctors in the same day, presenting a host of faked symptoms and picking up prescriptions for many drugs.
2. After filling the prescriptions with their Medicaid number, usually at zero cost to themselves, they sell them to a "noncon," a trafficker who doesn't deal in narcotics and is not usually under police surveillance.
3. The "noncon" then sells the prescription drugs back to a pharmacist at less than wholesale prices. The druggist then resells it to other Medicaid patients, once again billing the retail cost to the government— repeating the scam over and over.

The FBI launched an investigation of this racket in Illinois, where it has convicted fifteen individuals to date, including Medicaid patients, noncoms, and pharmacists. The probe is being extended nationwide.

The pharmacy end of the Medicaid racket has numerous scenarios. One of the boldest was pulled off in New Hampshire by what was advertised as "Your Hometown Pharmacy," the slogan of the Health Care Pharmacy, Inc. According to state investigators, they were found guilty of stealing $372,000 by billing for drugs that were never dispensed, and in some cases were not even prescribed. Dealing in expensive antibiotics like Cipro (five dollars a pill), they billed for 22,697 tablets even though they bought only 150 of the drug.

The Sonogram Scam

One racket that flourished for a while—and may still be going on in some communities—is the sonogram scam. A New York cabbie took the state Medicaid program for $140,000 by transporting (covered by Medicaid in most states) junkies from Harlem to his Queens apartment. The Medicaid "patients" would lie on a couch and for ten dollars would allow an ultrasound technician to take multiple sonograms using a portable machine.

The owners of a Bronx-based radiology billing company who were running the racket were indicted for stealing $335,000 from the state, failing to report over $10 million in Medicaid reimbursement on income tax returns, and paying large cash kickbacks—as much as seventy-five percent—to clinic owners and "salesmen" like the Queens cabbie.

Nothing is sacred to Medicaid cheats, not even pregnancy. A physician in Washington State ran a medical clinic specializing in abortions. A former employee of his blew the whistle, claiming that the doctor was cheating the government. He was served with a search warrant, during which the files of five hundred patients were taken for analysis by doctors in the fields of pathology, radiology, and gynecology.

What they learned was that the physician "regularly misstated the fetal age" of the embryo in order to collect more from Medicaid. Instead of billing the government for a first trimester abortion, he was upcoding the procedure by claiming that the woman was in her second trimester, which is a more complex operation. He even made false claims of headaches and infections in patients during follow-up visits in order to keep the lucrative scheme going.

Providers in the Medicaid program have even more opportunity to cheat than those handling Medicare. One reason, as we've seen, is that prescription drugs are covered—a $30-billion-a-year arena for fraud. On top of that, Medicaid usually insures the health of the mouth as well as the heart and lungs, something the taxpaying middle class can only dream of.

The Dental Racket

Some dentists salivate at the thought. Their fees are less than for private patients, but they know they're going to get paid. Secondly, there are virtually no restrictions of what they can provide. If a complex bridge costing $5,000 is needed for a seventy-year-old woman on welfare, so be it. The taxpayer, who may have missing teeth he can't afford to replace, will still—through his state and federal taxes—provide the woman with dental work, and the dentist with a prompt check.

Naturally, this $25-billion dental program includes anywhere from $5 billion to $10 billion worth of fraud and connivance, including the following:

- A Portland dentist was investigated by the Oregon fraud unit. A search warrant produced 2,900 Medicaid and private insurance records, while a probe of her garbage produced torn-up original bills and patient charts, showing large disparities. She pled guilty to theft by deception in the first degree, including submitting false claims to Medicaid and Blue Cross/Blue Shield.

- A New York dentist pled guilty to stealing $50,000 from Medicaid by upcoding his work, charging for periodontal scaling and root planing, which was either never provided or the work was of a simpler nature than his billing.

- A Pennsylvania dentist was sentenced to three years probation for a common fraud—billing personally for work done by unlicensed help. In this case, he was charged with billing for fluoride treatments done by others.

- In Florida, the Attorney General announced the arrest of two dentists and an office manager in the Clearwater office of Mobile Dental Health Service. A statewide grand jury delivered a 107-count indictment for "Medicaid Provider Fraud." Allegedly, while providing dental services for patients in a nursing home, they upcoded chair-side denture relines, falsely claiming they were done in a lab. In some cases they did no reline at all.

- Also in Florida, a dentist bilked the aged in nursing homes by billing Medicaid for dentures that were never provided. When they were, "they were of such poor quality that the recipient couldn't use them," says that state's Attorney General.

- A Boston dentist paid the government $195,000 in restitution and penalties for having billed Medicaid for "cosmetic" surgery, which is not covered by the government program.

- In New Jersey, the dentist-owner of Gentle Dental Care in Bridgeton was sentenced to four years in state prison for defrauding Medicaid by installing temporary crowns and billing for full noble metal ones.

- In New York City, a dentist was arrested for billing Aetna $3,462 for bridgework on a local public school teacher covered by the plan. There was only one problem with the claim: the patient had died three years before at the age of eighty-five.

These and other cases of fraud paint a portrait of our most honored professional—that of the medical practitioner—gone astray, of professionals preying on both the poor and aged, and, in the final analysis, on all taxpaying citizens.

What could be better than stopping the waste of $100 billion (at the very least) in medical, dental, and pharmaceutical fraud, and using the money for any good purpose, including lower federal taxes for all? And in the process, cleansing the stain that dishonest doctors have cast on the profession and, by extension, on their honest colleagues?

Solutions to the Fraud Crisis

Finding solutions is obviously a necessary goal. But has the situation worsened permanently? How can we possibly turn back the clock?

It may be considerably easier than skeptics think. To date, the government, the states, and private insurers have been lax in ferreting out the crooks. But beginning now, *if* we follow some logical guidelines, the fraud and the immorality of it all can be cut back. To accomplish this requires the participation of everyone involved—patients, doctors, medical employees, and the governments—local, state, and federal.

Here, then, are some things that we can do together to ferret out the medical crooks among us, and save a fortune in the process:

I. As a patient, examine your insurance statements carefully to see if costs have been exaggerated. Do not assume that they are correct. If you are suspicious, inquire of your doctor or the hospital and have them justify the charges. If you are not satisfied, call your insurer and tell them of any conflict. They might well investigate and find that you—and they—are being cheated. In the push toward HMOs, one-fourth of all patients are still covered by indemnity policies, with many thousands of cases of fraud each year.

II. If you are a Medicare patient, each visit prompts a statement from the government with the doctor's fee and how much they have allowed. Check that statement. If his fee is more than fifteen percent above the allowed amount, he is trying to cheat you and the government. They probably won't pay him the excess, but it might be a good indication of whether he is an honest doctor. If the amount of the bills seems high, but Medicare accepts it, it might mean he is upcoding. If you are truly suspicious, call the Medicare fraud hot line number (1-800-HHS-TIPS). You might get a good refund.

III. If, as a patient, you find that a doctor has been cheating either Medicare or Medicaid, don't stop there. It's probably a sign that he's cheating others as well. Demand that the government investigate his billing of other patients. It could develop into a large case with a sizable reward at the end.

IV. If you work in a doctor's office and you see evidence of upcoding, bundling, or procedures that were not performed on his bills to Medicare, don't feel any allegiance to your employer. Your obligation is to yourself as a taxpayer and to your nation. Become a whistle-blower and report him to the government. You will be doing your civic duty, and could receive a reward as well. The same is true of people who work in medical labs, nursing homes, home health care businesses, etc. You are not a "snitch," but a hero.

V. The investigations, which are now in the hands of the state fraud units, the FBI, and the Inspector Generals, have to become more centralized, with a common computer operation and joint task forces. At present, each group is doing too much of its own thing. A special bureau in the Department of Justice should be enlarged to handle the multiforce investigations. A good estimate is that less than ten percent of the medical fraud is currently being uncovered.

VI. The medical profession, which has not touched this problem with a ten-foot caduceus, has to become involved. This must go beyond lectures on ethics, to true disciplinary action. The AMA should set up its own enforcement unit, and have doctors call in with their suspicions of other doctors, which in turn should be relayed to government enforcement people. At present, some doctors are gaining a reputation for being less than honest, which in the long run rubs off on all members of the profession. Any member of a local medical society who has been "excluded" by Medicare or Medicaid should be kicked out of the AMA and reported to the state licensing authorities for disciplinary action, including the suspension, even removal, of his license to practice medicine.

As more insurers enter the picture and less out-of-pocket money is paid by patients, medical crooks feel more and more entitled to steal. Only by citizens letting the profession know that they are outraged will the fraud ever stop. The honored profession of medicine cannot support any more deviation from its dedication to the patient and honest practice.

Chapter IV
Medical Incompetence

The American Doctor:
Quality or Quackery?

The patient had just turned sixty-five and decided to get a thorough checkup. He had been feeling listless and wondered if his general practitioner could diagnosis the problem.

His blood test readings, taken in the morning before eating, were fine except for his sugar. The glucose level was too high. That number was 160, measured in milligrams per deciliter of blood, well above the normal level of 70 to 110.

"I'm afraid you probably have diabetes," the doctor told his patient. He scheduled a second reading to ensure its accuracy. "Yes, its still over 150, so I'm convinced you have Type Two, adult onset diabetes mellitus."

"Do I need to take insulin?" the nervous patient asked.

"No, not yet, anyway. We'll put you on a glyburide medication, which should help some."

The doctor explained that Type II diabetes, which usually starts after fifty, is quite different from juvenile diabetes, a malfunction of the pancreas in which the organ does not secrete enough insulin. Adult-onset diabetes strikes adults who are generally overweight, sedentary, older, and who have a history of the disease in the family. It affects people across the spectrum, but for some reason it affects Jews and Native Americans excessively, and sometimes blacks as well.

The problem with Type II diabetics—the most common group with the disease—is that for some largely unknown reason, their cells do not take up the insulin that is often produced in normal quantities. In some cases it can lead to the need to take insulin, but the doctor hoped that the sixty-five-year-old could manage his case with diet, exercise, and the drug.

The patient went along on this regimen for three years. His blood sugar levels were improved, but not fully controlled, going up and down. But he still felt weak from time to time, and woke up several times at night to urinate, a common symptom of diabetics.

At the end of the third year, his doctor moved elsewhere. A board-certified internist took over his practice. On the patient's first visit to the new doctor, he sat there as the doctor read his medical record and scowled.

"During all this time, didn't your previous doctor ever tell you to have your eyes examined by an ophthalmologist?"

"No. Why?"

Carefully, he explained that one of the side effects of diabetes is an eye condition known as diabetic retinopathy, in which the small blood vessels of the retina become damaged, causing decreased vision, which in many cases leads to blindness.

The frightened patient went to a local ophthalmologist, who gave him the bad news. He had already suffered damage in his retina. Fortunately, it was early in the deterioration and could be treated with laser surgery. If he was lucky, the damage could be slowed.

Was the patient's experience with his negligent first doctor unique?

A Doctor Is Not a Doctor Is Not . . .

Unfortunately not. Judging from careful studies, it appears that this type of negligence among physicians is *commonplace*. In this era of modern medical knowledge, one would think only a handful of physicians were ignorant—or careless—enough not to protect their diabetic patients, as much as possible, from eye damage.

Many people believe that, like Gertrude Stein's rose, a doctor is a doctor is a doctor.

If only that were so. Quality evaluations of physicians show that in no profession is there such a gap between the good and the incompetent, ignorant, or lazy practitioners. Lawyers, no matter how prosaic, can generally draw up wills or simple contracts. But it appears that medicine is quite different. The subject matter is not only more complicated and fast-changing, but the profession is dogged with legions of incompetent and insufficiently educated physicians who cause untold mayhem, as did the general practitioner with the diabetes patient.

In the case of diabetes, which now affects as many as 18 million Americans, proof of this enormous variation in doctor skill comes from an impressive study. Conducted by Dr. Jonathan P. Weiner of Johns Hopkins and his team, with the backing of the government's Office of Clinical Standards and Quality, it checked the treatment given to *every* diabetic Medicare patient in three states—Alabama, Iowa, and Maryland—who was treated by a primary care doctor: a general practitioner, a family physician, or a board-certified internist.

The results of this study of 97,000 patients were startling in a negative way. It appears that in the three vital procedures that every diabetic should receive, the researchers learned that on average the majority of doctors did not provide proper care.

The best measure of diabetic seriousness is not a transient measure of blood glucose done from time to time, but a test called "hemoglobin A1c," or "glycosylated hemoglobin," which measures the amount of sugar attached to blood over a period of six weeks.

Did the doctors take this essential measurement? No. The great majority failed to do it. *In fact, only sixteen percent of these primary care doctors did.*

What about the eye examination? *A majority of the diabetic patients did not receive it.*

Proper medical care of diabetics also requires that doctors check the cholesterol level of diabetic patients, who are much more prone to heart attacks than other people. Did doctors in this study do that simple test? *Almost half (forty-five percent) of the physicians did not screen their patients.*

The level of care was poor throughout. All three groups failed the test. And contrary to the belief that board-certified internists are particularly good family doctors, they did only a *bit* better than the G.P.s, belying their sometimes elevated reputation.

Says the report, in a masterpiece of understatement: "Elderly patients with diabetes do not appear to be receiving optimal care."

A Rise in Quality Studies

Quality studies that examine large numbers of patients are relatively new in medicine. More are being done today, including several like the diabetes study, which are financed by the government. The federal Office of Clinical Standards and Quality of HHS is footing the bill, which has already reached $250 million. According to Dr. Steven Jencks, director of that group, the work is done through a network of outside PROs, or Peer Review Organizations, a chain of fifty independent medical groups throughout the country. To date—since they were authorized in 1982—some one thousand studies have been completed or authorized.

How did the government get into the quality act? Because no one else was willing to do it. Fearful of insulting themselves or their colleagues, the AMA and local medical societies try to keep their dirty linen private, and maintain the illusion (almost David Copperfield–like) that a doctor is a doctor. But because Washington and the states spend $400 billion a year on Medicare and Medicaid, they have decided to check up and see how well doctors and hospitals are practicing medicine with our money.

The results are almost uniformly discouraging. In many, perhaps most, cases, the studies show that America's doctors are not up to the job of translating medical knowledge into uniform quality practice for their patients. For an industry that takes in over a trillion dollars a year, there are wide and dangerous gaps in standard care.

Failure in Treating Pneumonia

Another report backed by Medicare's Office of Clinical Standards and Quality dealt with an equally serious illness—pneumonia in the aged. Pneumonia accounts for more than 600,000 hospitalized cases a year among the aged, and overall is the sixth leading cause of death in the United States.

The researchers studied 14,069 patients over sixty-five years of age from across the nation who contracted the disease. They reported back in the *Journal of the American Medical Association* in late 1997. They were trying to learn if four vital procedures that could save the lives of the patients were done in time by physicians:

1. Administration of antibiotics within eight hours of hospital arrival
2. Taking a blood culture *before* administering the antibiotics, in the hope of getting an uncontaminated specimen
3. Taking a blood culture within twenty-four hours of arrival at the hospital

4. Assessing the patient's oxygenation within twenty-four hours of admission.

How did the doctors do?

In the first procedure, they failed in a quarter of all the cases.

In the second, the doctors' record was miserable. Almost half—forty-three percent—of the patients were not treated by their physicians with that quality standard.

In the third, the doctors failed one-third of the time.

The fourth was the only one with reasonable doctor performance, relatively speaking. Almost ninety percent of the patients were properly gauged for oxygenation—which still leaves a ten percent failure rate.

Overall, the performance of physicians in handling life-threatening pneumonia among senior citizens was poor. It was perhaps somewhat better than their work in diabetes, but philosophically worse, since they were dealing with an immediate life-threatening emergency. Their negligence, about which patients know nothing, is responsible for thousands of needless pneumonia deaths a year.

The failure of doctors to use acknowledged therapy has also resulted in perhaps thousands of needless deaths from Acute Myocardial Infarction (AMI), the classic heart attack.

In a sweeping study of heart attack victims published in *JAMA*, the Medicare records of 16,969 cases of AMI—every aged patient with the ailment discharged from the hospital in Alabama, Connecticut, Iowa, and Wisconsin for a nine-month period—were studied.

Did their doctors provide them with optimum therapy? Apparently not.

The investigators showed that many of the patients were undertreated, with often fatal results. Most cardiologists believe that beta-blockers should be administered to heart attack victims in order to prevent a second attack. These drugs, in use since the 1960s, slow the heart rate and reduce the force of the contraction of the heart muscle. In "ideal" patients, most academic physicians believe, the medication should be administered on discharge from the hospital.

But it was done in only less than half those cases, risking unnecessary future damage to the heart muscle and death itself.

The underuse of beta blockers by most doctors was confirmed in another study, this one done by the Harvard Medical School and the Harvard Pilgrim Health Care organization in Boston.

The research, which was also published in *JAMA*, covered 3,737 heart attack patients on Medicare in New Jersey. In the ninety days after discharge from the hospital, only one in five (21 percent) received beta-blocker therapy from their doctors. This was in spite of the fact that the same study showed that the death rate for those given the drug was 43 percent lower than for the others.

Overall, it is believed that the therapy increases the survival rate of heart victims by 20 to 40 percent. But these Medicare patients apparently were passed over by their doctors.

One of the nation's leading researchers is Dr. Robert H. Brook, professor of medicine at UCLA and senior investigator at the Rand Corporation. He has written extensively about quality studies, and comments on his own work as a young doctor in the emergency room of the Baltimore City Hospitals.

Dr. Brook did a follow-up study of a sample of patients six months after they had visited the emergency room. To his chagrin, he found the results of the medical activity was poor: "Professionals, myself included, believe in ourselves, and this belief can result in overestimation of our efficiency, efficacy, and effect." He found that of 141 sick patients, only a fourth received good care. In some cases it was the patients' fault, but the doctors failed as well.

More Discouraging Studies

Medical care has improved since then, and research studies on quality medicine have become more widespread and systematic. However, they are usually just as discouraging. In diplomatic academic language, Dr. Brook explains that we've learned "there are variations in the amounts of care and in the appropriateness and outcomes of care that we provide that are too large to be ignored."

He quotes studies that show that good preventive medicine is virtually ignored, even in our supposedly superior teaching hospitals. In sixteen academic primary care practices, for example, seventy percent of patients who should have received flu shots didn't get them.

Even after a vaccine was developed during World War II against certain stubborn strains of pneumonia-causing bacteria, it was not used extensively in the decades afterward, because doctors "assumed" that antibiotics would cure all pneumonias. As a result, thousands die each year of pneumococcal pneumonia caused by the *Streptococcus pneumoniae*, a deadly bacteria. The vaccine is excellent protection and generally lasts for life, but as Dr. Brook points out, four out of five of the surveyed doctors did not give it to their patients, even the vulnerable aged.

The Law: A Doctor Is a Doctor . . .

The startling aspect of our medical situation is that as far as the law is concerned, *a doctor is a doctor is a doctor*. As long as he has a license to practice medicine and perform surgery, he can legally do any procedure without any restraint. A general practitioner can even legally do brain surgery—if he can find a hospital to accommodate him.

This lack of regulation has even created a relatively new, and burgeoning, medical industry—surgery performed right in the doctor's office, a technique that threatens the quality of care.

For the last few decades, surgery has been somewhat monitored in the hospitals by peer review groups. But the quality clock is now being turned backward as physicians avoid the oversight of hospitals to do more cutting—and to use anesthesia—right in the office, out of the sight of anyone except the ignorant patient.

Just in one recent six-year period, according to Dr. Bernard Wetchler of the American Society of Anesthesiologists, the number of surgeries done in physicians' offices has tripled, from 400,000 to 1.2 million, with the trend growing.

Why? Because the cost-cutting revolution can destroy quality care. HMOs and other managed care companies are reducing costs by encouraging (and requiring) doctors to keep patients out of our expensive hospitals. By doing surgery in the office, says a Princeton Junction, New Jersey, doctor, physicians can earn part of the savings themselves. "In turn, physicians tell their patients, this will cost $1,500 in the hospital; $800 in the surgicenter [outpatient], or $300 in my office," says Dr. Ervin Moss. "Guess where the business is going?"

The problem, of course, is that doctors are not always good at administering anesthesiology. As a Connecticut anesthesiologist says: "A physician not familiar with his drugs can get in over his head."

One patient was undergoing surgery in the office of a dermatologist, who personally administered the anesthesia. He gave the patient a high dose of a drug called Midazolam. The patient reacted badly and was rushed to a hospital, where he slipped into a coma. Five weeks later he died of a heart attack.

It turns out that a healthy person might have survived the high dose of the anesthesia, but this patient was an alcoholic, something the dermatologist didn't learn about until after the operation. In a *good* hospital setting, a conference between the anesthesiologist and the patient is routine, something often avoided in the unsupervised office setting.

Many doctors know little about anesthesia or how to

resuscitate a patient—procedures others take care of in the hospital setting. Most doctors' offices don't even have such monitoring equipment as an oxygen ventilator meter or supplies to resuscitate a patient in an emergency. State regulation of in-office surgery is also quite lax in most states. Only Florida and a few other states now regulate sedatives and anesthesia in the doctor's office, a belated attempt to improve the situation.

Not only are most surgeries inadvisable in your doctor's office, but it now turns out that it is not the ideal place to have your blood or urine tested either. Two recent studies published in *JAMA* show that lab tests made by a physician or his staff are more likely to be incorrect than those done in larger independent labs and hospitals.

"If you don't have to, why should you take the chance?" says Dr. Lee Hilborne, a pathologist at UCLA.

Quality Care Can Be a Matter of Geography

Quality care sometimes depends not only on the doctor's ability, but where he—and you—live in the United States. Medical practice may be uniform in medical school, but that changes drastically, often for the worse, when doctors enter the real world.

Doctors typically fall into the medical habits and prejudices of the locality, much of it bad, even dangerous. This fact was conclusively proved by a massive study conducted by Dr. Mark Chassins, former New York State Health Commissioner, Dr. Brook, and others. It surveyed physician claims to Medicare from six states—Colorado, Iowa, Massachusetts, Montana, Pennsylvania, South Carolina—and Northern California.

The study involved 123 different medical and surgical procedures. It showed that in some communities, doctors use procedures excessively, as with unnecessary surgery, while in others there was too little medical intervention for the sick. The statistical work showed that the chances of the results being due to chance were in the order of

1,000 to one, not the kind of odds that will make you money in Las Vegas.

What did they learn?

- Coronary bypass operations per 100,000 Medicare beneficiaries varied from a low of seven to a high of twenty-three according to location.
- Electrocardiogram stress tests used to diagnose heart conditions were given to as many as 182 patients in some localities and only 49 in others.
- Shrinking hemorrhoids through injection was used on only one patient per 100,000 in one area but seventeen per 100,000 in another.

Other, smaller studies showed an even wider spread in what physicians *thought* was good medicine, a belief that varied from town to town in one region. A study of seven New England cities showed that by the time a man reaches eighty, the chance that his prostate will have been operated on by surgeons varies from twenty to sixty percent from town to town—hardly a statistic that indicates that doctors know what they're doing.

In the case of women, by the age of seventy the chances that she will have had a hysterectomy varied from one in five to almost four in five depending on in which city the doctors practiced.

Misplaced Confidence in Primary Doctors

A great deal of confidence is now placed on "primary doctors," probably to the detriment of quality care. The trend in medical colleges is toward training more family physicians and pediatricians rather than specialists and subspecialists, the type of physician that has made for superior clinical medicine.

As we've seen in the poor record of primary doctors in the treatment of Medicare patients with diabetes, this strategy is self-defeating. Most doctors did not perform eye examinations, while diabetic specialists (endocrinologists) routinely examine the eyes of patients or send them to an ophthalmologist.

The importance of specialists in quality care is also shown in the treatment of very sick children. Pediatricians are called specialists, but in reality they are primary care physicians for the young. However, there is a true pediatric specialist, a physician called a "pediatric intensivist," who is trained in the critical care of children.

When children are admitted to an Intensive Care Unit of a hospital, the presence—or absence—of a pediatric intensivist is closely tied to nothing less than survival or death.

This was confirmed by a massive study of 5,415 sick children in sixteen ICUs throughout the nation. Of that group, 248 of the children died. The study, which was conducted by several physicians including a group at the Department of Pediatrics of the George Washington School of Medicine, was published in *JAMA*.

What did it show? Simply that survival of the sick children was not based on the size of the ICU unit, the volume of admissions, or the public or private status of the hospital. However, as the authors show, "the relative odds of patient survival were 1.54 times higher in an ICU with a pediatric intensivist" than in an ICU without one. In layman's language, the chance of a very sick child living was often dependent on the specialist training of the person in charge, and not on the work of usual pediatricians.

Diagnosis is another massive challenge in achieving quality medical care, something at which many doctors fall far short. This includes not only "primary" doctors, but even specialists ostensibly highly trained in their work.

Misreading of Mammograms

One vital diagnostic tool is the mammogram, designed as an early screen to detect breast cancer. Once again, studies indicate the failure of physicians—in this case, radiologists—to perform as expected. At Yale University School of Medicine, researchers tried a simple test to gauge the accuracy of radiologists in reading mammogram plates. The guinea pigs were ten board-certified radiologists—seven in private practice and three academics—all experienced doctors who had previously evaluated thousands of mammograms.

They were given 150 mammogram plates, but were told nothing about the patient's medical history. Among the 150 mammograms were twenty-seven proven cases of cancer. Could the radiologists spot the malignancies?

Not particularly well, it turned out.

First, there wasn't much agreement among the ten radiologists. A report published in the *New England Journal of Medicine* showed that only in one case in fourteen did all the radiologists agree about what they saw. Among the twenty-seven cancer cases, only 54 percent of the time did the ten radiologists spot a mass, and only in 65 percent of the cancers were the radiologists suspicious enough to suggest a biopsy!

"Our results show that radiologists can differ, sometimes substantially, in their mammographic interpretations and recommendations for management," the report states unemotionally. "These results should not be regarded as casting doubt on the efficacy of mammography, the value of which has been well documented. *The variability found in this study, however, indicates that among radiologists who read mammograms, there is a wide range of accuracy.*"

An editorial in the same issue of the *New England Journal* said it best, if somewhat understated:

"It is disturbing that the interpreters failed to identify some patients with cancer."

Can anything be done to improve the early detection of breast cancer with mammograms? Yes. It seems that by using two *independent* radiologists to examine the same plate, lives can be saved. Although that is seldom done in regular practice, the concept was demonstrated in a study conducted at the University Hospital in Uppsala, Sweden. Two radiologists read each plate, but neither knew the name of the other radiologist or his conclusion. It was, in the parlance, a "blind" study.

The mammograms of 11,343 women aged forty-one to seventy-five were involved. Screeners found fifty-six breast cancers that they agreed upon. But *separately*, each of them found other cancers. One radiologist detected fourteen others, while the second physician found six. Together, through "double reading," they came up with seventy-six cancers, a fifteen percent improvement in detection.

How can a worried American woman patient duplicate this? Only by the time-honored method of seeking a *true* second opinion. This requires having another radiologist independently read the same plate *without giving him the name of the first radiologist or his diagnosis.*

Another problem in reading mammograms is the large number of "false positives" diagnosed by radiologists— cases in which doctors suspect a cancer that is not there.

A report from Harvard Pilgrim Health Care in Boston showed that such "false positives" are most common in women under fifty, and that a woman who has been taking an annual exam since age forty has a 50–50 chance of being incorrectly diagnosed for cancer over a ten-year period—plus a one in five chance of undergoing an unnecessary breast biopsy.

Misusing Stethoscopes

In the rushed environment of modern medicine, not only are modern diagnostic tools mishandled, but some patients and doctors are beginning to feel that the old-fashioned art of physical examination has somewhere been diminished, and with it the ability to properly diagnose ailments. A new study confirms that suspicion.

In *JAMA*, Dr. Salvator Mangione, who teaches the use of the stethoscope to medical students, reveals that young doctors in training are just no good at the vital art which can often detect problems in the heart and lungs. He studied the stethoscope skill of 453 residents from thirty-one different training programs in internal medicine. He found that their ability to identify common heart abnormalities was "disturbingly low."

His technique was simple: he had them listen to recordings of beating hearts, the same sounds they would hear with their stethoscopes, and asked them to diagnose any problems. Although he believes doctors should be accurate 70 to 80 percent of the time, *the medical graduates scored correctly in only 20 percent of the cases, missing four out of five abnormalities!*

Mangione believes that the residents' poor performance resulted from a lack of training. It seems that only a third of internal medicine residencies offer extensive training in "auscultation," the term for listening to the heart. It's especially disturbing, Dr. Mangione says, because he feels that 80 percent of a doctor's ability to diagnose illness stems from the medical history and the detailed physical examination.

Telling the Good Doctor from the Bad

The American patient is understandably confused, never really knowing if his doctor is good, bad, or indifferent. All he can gauge is the doctor's concern, warmth, and attention to his problems. But—and most patients do not understand this—they are very poor judges of their doctor's competence and the quality of his medical care.

Then who does know the truth?

The profession. But they're not talking. Most of that information is kept secret, as we shall see. Still, there are certain available, open clues that the patient can call on in choosing the right primary doctor or specialist:

1. Is he connected to a good, accredited hospital, with full privileges?
2. Even better, is he a full-time or part-time member of the faculty of a teaching hospital in the area? If a full-time academic and of mature age, is he at least an Assistant Professor? If in private practice, is he at least a Clinical Assistant Professor?
3. Does he have any special honors, such as having been "Chief Resident" during his residency? Did he belong to an honor society at medical college?
4. Did he attend a good medical school and not a college of osteopathy? While osteopaths (D.O., not M.D.) are licensed to practice medicine and surgery in almost all states, their schools generally have lower entrance requirements than traditional medical schools.
5. Have his peers honored him, including surveys taken by newspapers and magazines of the "best doctors," with other physicians doing the choosing?
6. Is he board-certified? Have you seen the credential on his wall? Is it from a legitimate accrediting organization?

Board Certification

Whether or not a doctor has his board certification in a particular specialty is an important piece of information. Unfortunately, by law, doctors can call themselves anything they wish, including "specialist" or "subspecialist."

Those without board certification often use euphemisms to confuse the public. A would-be orthopedist can merely say, quite legally, that his practice is "limited to orthopedics." Or a G.P. can label himself a "primary care specialist" and get away with it. A study of all "specialists" advertising in a Connecticut phone book showed that twelve percent of them did not have board certification.

The state has no control over what a specialist is or is

not, and cannot discipline any licensed physician for saying anything about his "specialty." It is the profession that controls specialties through the "boards," some forty in all. They are all accredited by the American Board of Medical Specialties (or the American Osteopathic Association, if you are so inclined). There is, in fact, no such designation as "general practitioner." If a primary care doctor has earned his "boards," it is either as a family physician, an internist, or a pediatrician in the case of children. G.P. just means that the physician has no recognized qualifications.

Are there many doctors without their boards? Upward of thirty percent, according to the AMA, or some 225,000 physicians. What should the patient make of this large group of doctors? There are several possibilities:

- They applied for their boards but flunked the examination. Most specialties allow the doctor to take their test three or four times over a period of five or six years. In ten specialties, however, doctors can take the test an unlimited number of times until they pass—or give up.
- They have decided not to apply for their boards. Since it is a voluntary action, these physicians will have to deal with hospitals, HMOs, and patients who will probably ask them, "Why not?"
- They have never taken a residency in an American or Canadian hospital, a qualification for board certification.
- They might be older doctors who began practice when the boards were not very important, and feel incapable of passing the tests today. Or don't care anymore.

Some physicians who are not board-certified try to dodge the issue by calling themselves "board-eligible." However, in recent years most specialty boards have made such a designation unethical.

Watch Out for the Inferior Boards

Some physicians who have failed the boards of regular credentialing organizations—American College of Surgeons, American Board of Internal Medicine, etc.—are making end runs around the conventional wisdom. They are taking their boards with a new fringe group that seems suspiciously inferior.

That organization comes out of Las Vegas, Nevada, and is called the "American Federation of Medical Accreditation." It accredits not only accepted medical specialties, but some flamboyant new ones, including *bionic rehabilitative psychology, ringside medicine and surgery, percutaneous dissectomy*, and *radio-frequency surgery*.

A spokesperson for the regular boards is contemptuous of the new group. "We feel board certification should involve training with certain standards. If someone passes an exam given by one of our member boards, the public can be sure that the doctor has met those standards."

The new boards don't always require hospital training in the specialty field, as do conventional boards. They deal with thousands of doctors left out of the present system for one reason or another. Some of the physicians have flunked their regular boards. Others, as New York neurosurgeon Rafael Cilento claims, have been discriminated against. He cites the case of a neurosurgeon who took his residency at Henry Ford Hospital, an excellent institution, then passed the specialist written exam. But he believes this doctor was blocked from taking the orals for board certification because of a personal conflict with his residency program director.

Surely such cases exist. And there is *true* discrimination in board certification against foreign-trained doctors, who cannot even apply if they have not taken a residency in an American or Canadian hospital.

But barring facts that truly excuse the absence of the credential, the patient is safest by insisting that his doctor be board certified by a traditional specialty organization.

These qualifications and information about a doctor's background and training are easily available through two directories found in most public libraries. One is the *Directory of Physicians in the United States*, and the second is the *Official ABMS Directory of Board Certified American Medical Specialists.*

The AMA has put its file of 650,000 doctors onto the World Wide Web, and you can call up the basic positive information by accessing: http://www.ama-assn.org. Once you've called that up, follow through to "Physician Select."

Checking out specialists is just as easy. Merely call 1-800-776-2378 to confirm that he (or she) is truly board certified.

The Code of *Omerta*

But what you won't find in your library is the possible hidden side of a physician's background. That a particular doctor may be incompetent or untrustworthy is generally known only to the profession, which keeps it secret from the public. The profession operates under a strict code of *omerta*, a conspiracy of silence that protects fellow doctors and purposely keeps patients in the dark.

What the patient should know about a doctor, but usually doesn't, includes the following:

- Has he ever been denied hospital privileges anywhere in the United States at any time in his career?
- Has he ever been kicked out of a hospital, that is, had his privileges taken away?
- Has he taken a board certification test and failed? How many times?
- Has he been permanently barred from board certification?
- Does he have a history of malpractice lawsuits? Was he vindicated or did he lose? Or did his insur-

ance company have to make a settlement with the injured patients?

- Has the state licensing board heard charges against him for incompetence? Did they decide in his favor or against him?
- Has he been disciplined by the state for poor professional practices, such as inappropriate sexual behavior with patients, lying on applications, fraud, or other violations of the Hippocratic Oath?
- If a surgeon, is he prone to unnecessary surgery, either because of ignorance or to line his pocket?
- Has he been charged, or admitted, or convicted of drug abuse or alcoholism?
- Has his license to practice medicine ever been suspended? And for how long? And in your state or elsewhere?

The fear of being charged with a violation is so frightening to doctors that the profession usually closes ranks when one of their own is being threatened. That's when the code of silence comes into play, often to the great detriment—even professional ruin—of anyone who would blow the whistle on an offender.

A Case of Intimidation

This happened to a registered nurse who worked in the Intensive Care Unit of a hospital. Her six-year-old female patient was in a light coma, which meant she could feel pain but was unconscious. All her young life, the child suffered from a seizure disorder that was partially controlled by anticonvulsant drugs. But the remedy had taken a toll on her liver, which doctors believed caused her coma. However, the child was in no immediate danger while she waited in hope for a liver transplant.

Under orders form a kidney consultant on the case, the nurse performed a hemoperfusion to cleanse the blood of the anticonvulsant drug. All seemed well, and the nurse left the child in stable condition in the ICU. Two days later the consultant passed her in the hall, sadly informing her of the child's death not long after a kidney dialysis he had ordered.

The nurse was shocked. The child's kidneys were healthy and dialysis was surely not called for. It turned out that the doctor had ordered the dialysis to lower the high sodium level of her blood. It was an extreme, unnecessary, and dangerous measure for a lesser problem, with grave potential danger, especially for patients with healthy kidneys. The doctor had made a fatal error.

The hospital administrator warned the nurse not to talk about the case to anyone—that they needed "damage control" or they'd be in "big trouble." To save her job, she decided to say nothing, but to salve her conscience, she offered to lecture on sodium control during dialysis, the action that had killed the child.

Immediately, she was marked as a potential security risk. No one would talk to her, and she was transferred from dialysis to orthopedics. No one in the hospital ever discussed the death of the child. The nurse did finally become a whistle-blower, in a way, by writing an article on this case of obvious medical malpractice. But still intimidated by the professional code of silence, she disguised the names of the patient, the doctor—and herself.

The medical code of *omerta* not only requires silence about the errors and fraud of other doctors, but applies to the physician himself. Few doctors step up to the metaphorical plate to announce that yes, they have been guilty of malpractice. They generally refuse to admit that despite their best efforts to heal their patients, that they have erred and caused grave harm.

When a doctor makes a mistake that could lead to a malpractice suit, the first thing his insurance company tells him is to keep his mouth shut, not to discuss the case with his patient, or with anyone.

But a leading physician has now asked doctors to be straightforward and admit all their mistakes—up front and early. Writing in the *Journal of General Internal Medi-*

cine, Dr. Albert Wu, associate professor of the School of Public Health in Baltimore, reveals that doctors usually keep serious mistakes to themselves, which he feels is itself an error. Previously, he published a study showing that the habit starts early. Among doctors in training at three large teaching hospitals, only half of them discussed mistakes with senior doctors. Only a quarter of the young physicians told the truth to their patients and family.

Wu says that the truth is always the best route. First, it is the moral thing to do, especially since the doctor's first responsibility is to act in the patient's interest. Secondly, the patient should be told so that remedies can be openly attempted. Third, the patient may deserve compensation—in money—for the mistake.

Another reason is that doctors who cause harm inadvertently often suffer from guilt, which can be purged by telling the truth. It's even possible that the truth, which builds faith in the doctor's integrity, could forestall a malpractice suit.

Naturally, the insurance companies firmly disagree. A spokesman for the Physicians Insurers Association of America said Dr. Wu's admonition was like asking doctors to "commit professional suicide."

So until medicine becomes an open, honest profession, one can expect more and more malpractice suits, and with it, the patients need to know who is committing the mistakes.

As the result of the 1986 Health Care Quality Improvement Act, all the available negative information about doctors—at least those resulting from official action—has been catalogued in a nationwide computerized file called the National Practitioners Data Bank, which has been established by the federal government.

The data bank includes the names, full background, and liabilities of those physicians and other health practitioners who have had:

- Their licenses suspended for thirty days or more
- Disciplinary action of any kind taken by state licensing boards

- Disciplinary action or restrictions put on by hospital peer review committees
- Adverse action by specialty boards
- Adverse action against their hospital privileges
- Malpractice cases in which settlements have been made or the cases lost by practitioners.

The data bank, which was started in 1991, is operated by Unisys in Virginia for the federal government. The bank now has 118,000 practitioners on its computer rolls—85 percent doctors and 15 percent dentists—all of whom have been in some sort of professional trouble. As of the end of 1997, according to Dr. Thomas C. Croft, who as director of the Division of Quality Assurance of the HHS, runs the operation, there were 176,000 reports of actions against practitioners in the bank, 136,000 of which involved malpractice suits.

The remainder of the reports involve adverse disciplinary actions controlled by state licensing boards. These were actions against health professionals who have lost their hospital privileges or had their licenses to practice suspended or terminated.

Watch Out for Multiple Offenders

Some doctors have had multiple charges against them. About 4,500 physicians have been subject to both adverse disciplinary actions by states *and* lost or settled malpractice suits. Another 1,100 have been involved in adverse disciplinary actions and "excluded" from Medicare or Medicaid programs.

That last number will soon become much higher. The Medicare and Medicaid exclusion listings on the data bank began only recently with the passage of the Health Insurance Portability and Accounting Act of 1996, generally referred to as the Kassebaum-Kennedy Bill. But the names of "excluded" doctors will be entered from now on.

All these names of physicians and other health providers—including dentists, osteopaths, chiropractors, and podiatrists—eventually end up in the National Practitioners Data Bank, together with information on malpractice cases submitted by insurance companies and self-insured physicians and dentists. Under the law, passed in 1986 and later amended (Title IV of Public Law 99–660), state licensing authorities are required to report any licensure or disciplinary activity to the bank. Hospitals and other credentialing bodies *must* query the data bank before granting privileges for the first time, and when renewing credentials. They must also make queries to the bank every two years about their existing staffs. It states:

"The intent of this legislation . . . is to improve the quality of medical care by encouraging physicians . . . to identify and discipline those who engage in unprofessional behavior; and to restrict the ability of incompetent(s) . . . to move from state to state without disclosure of the practitioners' previous damaging or incompetent performance."

Most entries on the NPDB come from the state licensing boards, whose disciplinary activity is on the rise. In 1996, according the Federation of State Medicial Boards, there were 4,400 cases involving errant doctors, a number that rises each year. Any actions taken to suspend or take away licenses, or to put doctors on probation, are sent out from one state to another over Boardnet, which connects twenty-nine state boards, and are also given to the national group.

How can the public access the damaging information?

They can't. The national data bank, which includes all malpractice cases in America, is available to health providers (for three dollars a name), but the record of offending doctors is absolutely closed to those who have the greatest need to know: Mr. and Mrs. John Q. Public.

What about disciplinary actions taken by states? That is also catalogued on the data bank, but is equally unavailable to the patient. The same is true of the lists compiled by the Federation of State Medical Boards, which has a national roster of medical discipline cases going back many years—also open only to hospitals, HMOs, and other professional groups.

The patient can *sometimes* learn about a doctor's checkered past from his state government. The information is not truly open, but a person can ask his state's medical licensing board for information on a particular doctor. Some states will honor the request, but others will only reluctantly give out the information if the patient files a Freedom of Information request. (Check your own state.)

The Public's Need to Know

There is a battle raging over patient access to this national font of information. Health activists, including Dr. Sidney Wolfe of the advocacy group Public Citizen in Washington, want the files opened to the public. Senator Ron Wyden, democrat of Oregon, whose bill established the NPDB in the first place, has proposed legislation to open the files of "repeat offenders," those doctors who have lost or settled several malpractice cases. But thus far he has failed to convince Congress.

"It's hard to believe," Senator Wyden says, "that right now Americans are granted more information when purchasing a breakfast cereal than when choosing a heart surgeon."

"Senator Wyden's first bill, in 1994, never got out of committee," Dr. Thomas Croft explained when interviewed. "His second bill, which was co-sponsored by Senator Olympia Snowe of Maine, did reach the floor but it was voted down. Had it passed, the data on doctors—including information on malpractice cases—would have been published and distributed to public libraries so that patients could check out doctors. But Wyden's bill was not just about that access. It also included material on gag rules for HMOs, and it was defeated."

Dr. Croft expects that some compromise will eventually be reached on disclosure, and that it might affect only "repeat offenders," as Senator Wyden has suggested.

Meanwhile, a handful of states are not waiting for the federal government. Massachusetts was the first state to set up an information system on doctors for the general public. In November 1996 its Physician Profile Law took effect, and is now in full operation. Any citizen can ask for a medical "report card," a full profile of up to ten licensed Massachusetts doctors, and will receive a package containing information on their training, hospital affiliations, awards and publications, plus what was usually just whispered about: a full record of malpractice cases they lost or settled, plus any disciplinary action taken by the state or a hospital.

"The program has been a great success," says a spokesman for the state medical registry. "We've had 87,000 requests for physician profiles along with 2.5 million hits on our web site. All of our records are on the Internet and available to everyone."

(Internet users can peek in on Massachusetts physicians by calling up the web page www.docboard.org)

Other states, including Florida and Rhode Island, are considering joining Massachusetts in becoming "patient friendly."

Meanwhile, Dr. Croft's organization is starting still another data bank on doctors and other providers. Called the "Fraud and Abuse Data Bank," it was launched in March 1998, and will combine information from the Justice Department, the state fraud agencies, Medicare, and the Inspector General's Office of HHS into one computer list.

But once again, this vital bank of information will not be open to the long-suffering American public.

Disclosure of Malpractice Cases

The AMA, of course, is always more protective of doctors than of their patients. It is adamantly against all disclosures to the public, and even wants all revelations about malpractice cases taken out of data banks. They believe that such information is not only inappropriate, but often misinterpreted by patients. The AMA believes that lost malpractice suits are not necessarily evidence of bad care.

Right now, doctors are allowed to enter a hundred-world "rebuttal" into the record, their statement of what they think actually took place in a malpractice suit they lost, or settled. But AMA people think this is insufficient, claiming that consumers could be misled into believing that a doctor who has lost a malpractice suit, or even two, is less able to practice good medicine.

They point out that factors such as geography (more malpractice suits in the Northeast and the West Coast) and the doctor's specialty come into play. For instance, says the AMA, eighty percent of the ob/gyn doctors have been sued at least one time, and most more than once.

At the same time, small settlements are often paid to plaintiffs by insurance companies just to get rid of so-called "nuisance suits" which would be expensive to defend. To protect against these cases going into the data bank, says the AMA, a $50,000 settlement should be the threshold payment before the data is recorded. As of now, all malpractice settlements are recorded, no matter how small.

During one AMA meeting, delegates asked that the NPDB be disbanded and replaced by a nationwide depository run by the Federation of State Medical Boards, the people responsible for local discipline. As far as the AMA is concerned, the only pertinent data are education, training, specialty, conviction for violent crimes, adverse licensing decisions, or actions by hospital boards.

Dr. Croft admits there is the danger of statistical confusion when reporting malpractice judgments or settlements. Of the thousands of doctors who've lost cases, sometimes the bank records the same case several times—based on several separate payouts.

Dr. Lynn Softer of Public Citizen, who is on the bank's executive committee, believes otherwise. She has said that the technical problems can be handled. What is at stake, she believes, is the right of consumers to know more about their doctors.

To make an end run around various government activities and the medical profession's infighting, Public Citizen publishes a volume entitled *16,638 Questionable Doctors*, an index to physicians who have been in trouble with the licensing boards for one reason or another. The four-volume national edition costs $307.50, but you can find it in some libraries. Individual state reports cost $23.50, and they can be ordered by calling 1-800-588-7780.

"Many state medical boards and other regulatory agencies," states Dr. Sidney M. Wolfe, project director on the book, "have either entirely failed to catch doctors guilty of incompetence, drunkenness, or patient abuse, or have let them get away with slaps on the wrist such as fines or reprimands."

AMA Starts Doctor Accreditation

The quality battle is heating up and will be the major field of medical infighting for the next decade or more. The latest entrant is a new form of accreditation of doctors. This is being run by the AMA, which is deathly afraid that unless they do it, some group less friendly to doctors will.

Right now, after receiving his license to practice medicine and surgery in all fifty states, there is no physician accreditation that involves all doctors. The specialties award "board certification," but some 225,000 doctors don't have it.

The AMA wants to add their certification to the doctor's credentials. In 1998 the program was first put into effect in New Jersey, where applications for accreditation are coming in. "The program is voluntary, and we farm out to organizations the surveying and grading of the doctors," an AMA spokesman explained.

Whether or not the AMA will be truly strict in their accreditation program or whether it will be a stamp of approval handed out willy-nilly is yet to be shown. If precedent is the rule, it will be a flexible, permissive operation, in which all doubts will be settled in favor of the physicians. After all, the AMA has always functioned as a doctor union, much like the teacher's NEA.

Solutions to the Quality Crisis

Data banks, accreditations, and the public's access to information about all doctors are important in elevating the quality of medical care. Yet the real problem is that most doctors, as we have seen, do not practice uniformly good medicine.

The villain here is the absence of standards of quality care. Even where they do exist—in the best educated segments of the profession—they are not properly disseminated to practitioners, who operate independently.

Because of the absence of *uniform* standards of quality, each doctor tends to reinvent medicine as he goes along, grabbing a piece of information here and there and putting it all together in an ad hoc, often unscientific approximation of medical science, which may or not may not conform to what the profession knows.

As a result, the patient can seldom be sure the correct procedures are being used on his behalf. The doctor's methods may be wrong, they may be incomplete, they may be outdated, but the patient has no way of knowing this. The patient's recourse—only after bad treatment—is a malpractice suit, which is hardly compensation for a serious iatrogenic injury.

What we need in order to ensure quality care is an entirely new professional mind-set, one that will develop *specific routine guidelines of what is expected of every doctor in the diagnosis and treatment of specific ailments.*

The absence of specific guidelines produces an enormous—and dangerous—variance in treatment. This was shown by a study of pneumonia cases that patients picked up in the community and not in the hospital. Though medical protocols indicate that it's necessary for doctors to take both sputum and blood cultures as soon as patients come into the hospital through the emergency room, it was done in as few as 36 and 53 percent of the time respectively!

In this study, a quality improvement team in New Jersey tried to change the situation by setting up guidelines for doctors and having them enforced. For example, antibiotics were not being administered rapidly enough because of professional diplomacy. The doctors in the hospital felt that *the patient's community doctor had to be contacted before they began treatment.* This touch of traditional courtesy only resulted in more pneumonia deaths. The quality team finally decided to treat the patient first and worry about the sensibilities of the patient's outside doctor later on.

Deming's Quality Control Method

We are reminded by quality-conscious physicians that the "theory of knowledge" is all-important. That was developed by W. Edward Deming, the man who brought quality control to Japan soon after World War II, and who is credited with that nation's industrial success. "In medicine," say two researchers at Case Western Reserve University School of Medicine, "this means applying the scientific method to everyday work. . . ."

This is easier said that done. But in one case outlined in the treatment of community-acquired pneumonia, the mortality rate was cut from ten percent to seven percent, along with the saving of many lives. They accomplished this by developing strict guidelines for treatment—standing orders that had to be obeyed. They tested their theories, then *institutionalized* them.

Most doctors don't like being told that their procedures are not good enough. However, virtually all studies show that in many, perhaps most, cases, they are not.

Thus, the patient today must understand that *he* himself is personally the key to quality medical care. He must know where to look, and must be sufficiently aware of his own condition and the latest in medical treatment if he is to become the *successful* patient. In a way, he must be the capital of his medical ship, the supervisor of his own health. He must not be willing to leave his fate to anyone, willy-nilly, without confidence that the treatment is the correct one.

To accomplish this, he must study his ailment in depth and become, in some ways, almost as conversant with the situation as are doctors. This is one reason (the baby boomers turning fifty is another) why bookstore health sections have grown tremendously in recent years, with whole publishing imprints now dedicated to helping the layperson understand diseases, conditions, pharmaceuticals, homeopathic remedies, etc. Indeed, most new drugs or supplements put on the market inspire several books on their pros and cons.

There are two books which I have found particularly useful. The first is the *Merck Manual of Medical Information, Home Edition*, 1,509 pages of detailed descriptions and available treatments (including the newest) of virtually every ailment, written by the nation's leading specialists. It is published by Merck and available in most book stores. Or you can write to the Merck Publishing Group, Rahway, New Jersey.

The second is a series of "White Papers" on some thirteen different ailments written by the faculty of Johns Hopkins Medical College. The booklets, which are generally seventy pages in length, offer even greater detail than the *Merck Manual* on the diagnosis and treatments of such common problems as diabetes, heart disease, hypertension, arthritis, and prostate trouble as well as an essay on longevity. They are available for $19.95 each from Johns Hopkins Medical Institutions, Subscription Department, Box 420083, Palm Coast, Florida, 32142.

Intensive research on one's ailment can also be conducted by the patient by using the public library, concentrating on articles published in *JAMA* and the *New England Journal of Medicine*, the two quality general medical journals. Indexes to both are usually available in the better libraries.

Once armed with knowledge, the patient is better able to evaluate his doctor's diagnosis, treatment, and prognosis. In serious ailments, we assume this also includes a second opinion—*totally independent of the first.* This requires the patient's ability to be secretive: not to divulge the name or the recommendations of the first doctor to the second. Some patients might find that three independent opinions are of even greater value.

Once armed with medical consensus plus one's own education on the subject, the patient should be prepared to act. However, in some cases, conventional medical opinion is not always sufficient, especially in cases of life or death.

Take one case of cancer, in which *several* physicians concluded that the patient's chances of survival were nil. What the patient, Gregory White Smith, was told by doctors was that his brain tumor was inoperable and that he had only three to six months to live. But one day, Smith, a successful writer, went to a dinner party given by television luminary Phil Donahue. At the party he sat next to actor and talk show host Charles Grodin, who told him about his own battle to save his ex-wife from breast cancer. "No one's got the last word," Grodin told Smith.

Encouraged, Smith kept talking to other doctors until he found one willing to give him an "experimental" treatment. The result, some eleven years later, is that the tumor is partially gone. He still suffers from numbness and partial deafness, but he is alive. In fact, Smith is active in a new business. As co-author of the directory, *The Best Doctors in America,* he is helping people find the right physician for them. He has personally helped 3,000 patients find doctors, earning a fee of anywhere from $50 to $500 for each.

Not every patient will be involved in such a life and death equation, but the nation and the medical profession must become more compulsive about providing quality care. Here, then, is a list of general rules that the profession should follow to raise the quality of medicine practice:

I. Stricter enforcement of discipline by removing the licenses of doctors who do not measure up. The criteria? Good medical standards, to be enforced by peer groups, other doctors who are unafraid to face up to the incompetence of colleagues.

II. Recertification of *all* medical licenses by the states through regular examinations every seven years, tests that doctors will have two chances to pass. If not, their license to practice should be suspended, then after appeal, removed. Such actions should be coordinated among all states so that failing doctors cannot simply move their practices elsewhere.

III. Continuing education is now a lax procedure, with most doctors merely attending a certain number of conferences in order to keep their hospital privileges. This must be transformed into a formal educational program. County and state medical societies should require that *all* doctors attend classes at local medical colleges at least ten days a year, taking graded exams offered by the schools.

IV. To make the practice of medicine more *uniform*, all specialty boards should issue detailed guidelines on the minimum treatment of diseases, from arthritis to coronary disease, that doctors should follow in handling their patients. These guidelines should also be sent to primary doctors, and be shared with their patients, who can check if they have been carried out in their cases.

V. All doctors should be required, by state law, to be board certified. They should be given three chances to pass their respective boards, or have their licenses revoked after appeal. In the case of primary doctors, they can receive board certification as family physicians, internists, or pediatricians.

VI. State laws should be changed to make it illegal for doctors to fudge a lack of board certification. Doctors should no longer be allowed to use such phrases as "practice limited to cardiology," or "board eligible," a common obfuscation. The only exception might be older doctors, who will be "grandfathered" for a certain period of time.

VII. County and state medical societies should establish audit units that make random checks of practicing physicians to see if they are practicing quality medicine. The audit personnel should be doctors from other areas, who will not be influenced by local biases or friendships. Failure to pass an audit and a repeat reexam should be entered in the doctor's record in the National Practitioners Data Bank. Consistent failure should result in removal of the license to practice medicine.

VIII. The National Practitioners Data Bank should be opened to the public on the following basis: all disciplinary and adverse actions against a doctor should be published regularly and distributed through public libraries. The data bank should also include the names of doctors who have failed the specialty boards three times. In the case of malpractice, the names of doctors who have lost or settled two or more cases should be published, along with the physician's rebuttal.

IX. The new fraud data bank being developed by the government should also be made public, including those practitioners who have been "excluded" from Medicare and Medicaid.

Medical quality is surely not something we can leave to the individual doctor, who often has an idiosyncratic view of medicine, one which may—or may not—jibe with the best scientific standards of the profession.

To protect the patient and ensure that he or she receives the best possible care, we must not only be sure they are properly insured, but properly cared for medically. This requires considerably more attention to medical competence—by the profession, the law, and the sophisticated patient.

Chapter V

Unnecessary Surgery

The Knife and You

In Massachusetts, a pregnant mother who happened to be a nurse was looking forward to the delivery of her fifth child. She was proud that despite the fashion of cesarean births, all four of her children were delivered traditionally. She expected the same this time.

But when she was almost ready to give birth, her obstetrician suddenly surprised her. He was going on vacation and might not be at her bedside when she was ready to deliver. Instead, he told the woman, he had scheduled her for a cesarean.

The woman protested. Being a nurse, she knew that a C-section, as it is often called, was a serious surgical operation. An incision cuts through the abdomen to the uterus in order to reach the child. Besides, she had given birth to four children vaginally and didn't want a cesarean. The doctor became furious with her, angrily conjuring up dire images of "her uterus blowing up like a hydrogen bomb."

The woman finally relented, and while her obstetrician was on vacation, the on-call substitute doctor performed the operation.

As a result of the surgery, the woman developed intestinal obstructions, which led to several more operations, including the loss of some of her intestines. She spent two years in the hospital and in bed, then sued the obstetrician. The verdict was in her favor, with a judgment of $1.5 million.

Was the C-section necessary? Probably not. And in that, the injured woman has plenty of company.

In 1997, there were some four million live births. Of these, 23 percent were delivered by cesarean operation. In contrast, in 1970—before the procedure became fashionable—only 5.5 percent of births were by cesarean. The female anatomy has not changed in thirty years, but 920,000 cesarean births are now performed each year, making it the most common major surgery in America.

Why the fourfold increase in such surgeries? The answer, of course, is that the C-section is caught up in the epidemic of unnecessary surgery that plagues American medicine and assaults every organ of its often hapless patients.

Each year, like our nurse, 25 million Americans go under the knife, fully confident that their surgeons are following one of the most important medical credos—*Primum Non Nocere*, or, "First Do No Harm." Every patient is made to believe that his surgery is necessary, the risks acceptable, and the exorbitant costs fully justified.

Unfortunately for millions each year, this may not be the case. They may instead be victims of powerful medical propaganda that makes *every* operation seem essential. But the reality is that unnecessary surgery, whether performed by doctors who operate out of ignorance, self-delusion, or simple greed has long plagued medicine and today still reaches epidemic proportions.

Unnecessary surgery has been examined, ridiculed, and insulted. Yet it still exists. So it is important for the patient to know as much as he can about which operations are good and appropriate and which are not. It is not an easy decision, but one the profession—and its patients—must make.

Old Standby: T & A Surgery

For almost a century, American surgeons enriched themselves by operating on harmless tissue. Many a doctor paid for his bread-and-Buicks with the old standby of "T & A"—removal of the tonsils and adenoids. You might think this a practice of the past. Actually, despite continuous criticism that most tonsillectomies are medically unnecessary, it is still one of the most common operations in America. Each year, 400,000 children go under the knife to remove what are mostly harmless—even valuable—tonsils at the back of the throat, in what has been described as "an American ritual."

According to *Clinical Reference Systems*, as many as thirty percent of children in some communities undergo a T & A even though "only two or three percent of children have adequate medical indications for this procedure." Translated into lay language, it means that *most* tonsillectomies are an unwanted invasion of the body.

Besides, it is not harmless surgery, as some parents might think. Some twenty-five children die each year as a result of the operation, and two thousand children bleed on the fifth to eighth postoperative day, requiring a blood transfusion or additional surgery. In some cases, children develop "hypernasal" speech because the soft palate no longer closes completely.

Tonsils are not, as some believe, vestigial organs without a purpose. Tonsils produce antibodies that fight nose and throat infections and also confine the infection to the throat, stopping it from spreading to the neck or bloodstream. If they become infected, the standard procedure is ten days of antibiotic treatment. Seldom is it necessary to excise them. Once that is done, their valuable antibody function is over.

Parents worry about "large" tonsils, normal during childhood, which reach their peak size between the ages of eight and twelve, after which they shrink. They are only too large if they touch each other. Some surgeons claim that removal of the tonsils will decrease the number of upper respiratory infections, but that is more folklore than science. The same is true of "strep throat," which should be treated with antibiotics unless the child has seven or more such infections each year. Then perhaps the tonsils should be surgically removed.

Adenoids Are Also Sacrificed

The argument for removal of adenoids is equally specious. Once it was believed that the surgery would open the eustachian tube and reduce the number of ear infections. New research shows this is not the case.

So when is surgery necessary? In the case of adenoids, persistent nasal obstructions, severe snoring and mouth breathing due to large adenoids can be reasons for surgery. In the case of tonsils, experts say there *are* some conditions that call for tonsillectomy, including reduced breathing that cuts down blood oxygen and can even cause heart failure. Another reason is that the tonsils are so enlarged that they interfere with swallowing, especially in children with especially small mouths. The most serious reasons are deep abscesses and tumors in the tonsils.

But, warn experts, this does not happen 400,000 times a year. So parents should be sure—perhaps with a second opinion—before their children's tonsils and adenoids are routinely excised. More than likely the operation is unnecessary.

Unnecessary Appendectomies

Appendectomies are another standard item in the surgeon's inventory. Years ago there was an epidemic of such operations, but as doctors have learned how to better diagnosis "appendicitis," the number has been reduced. However, there are still 250,000 appendectomies performed each year, and professionals estimate that 50,000 are unnecessary.

Why? First, it's important to understand why surgeons sometimes cut out the appendix. The organ is a small, finger-shaped tube projecting from the large intestine near the point where it joins the small intestine. It is believed that the appendix has some immune function in the body, but it's not clear what it is.

In some patients, generally between the ages of ten and thirty, the organ becomes inflamed and infected. If it is not treated, it can rupture and cause peritonitis in the abdomen, which is a life-threatening disease. To avoid that, surgeons often remove the organ when a patient has severe abdominal pain.

The problem is that diagnosis is not easy. In fact, after surgery, about twenty percent of the removed appendixes turn out to be normal. Sometimes the error is the result of poor diagnosis by the surgeon—that the pain originated in another, unknown source. Other times, it is because some surgeons tend to be too quick with the knife.

A new diagnostic technique might reduce these unnecessary operations. Radiologists from the Massachusetts General Hospital believe they have developed an accurate way of diagnosing acute appendicitis: a special spiral scanning technique directed *only* at the region of the appendix in place of the standard CAT scan. And instead of the usual method of infusing the opaque dye by mouth or intravenously, they inject it directly into the colon. The result is a clearer picture of the appendix, and thus a better diagnosis.

Their six-month study of one hundred patients diagnosed

with appendicitis produced only two "false positives," patients who did not have the disease. This is in contrast to the twenty percent proven to have healthy appendixes *after* surgery. The technique, called "Focused Appendix CT" or FACT, could eliminate this type of unnecessary surgery—at least in the hands of honest surgeons.

Unlike other doctors, surgeons are not content to live on forty dollars per patient visit. Many still see the operating table as a chance for the brass ring—the new SL600 Mercedes coupé for $139,000, or even the down payment on a piece of land in Southampton or Malibu.

Surgery is the *big business* of the medical business, the only way a physician can reach the seven figure ($1,000,000) a year income.

"It's not fair," says a Connecticut board-certified internist. "I can work for days on end to save a pneumonia patient, getting a pittance per hour from Medicare. Meanwhile, not far from me in the hospital, a surgeon is operating on someone and taking home five thousand dollars for a morning's work. No doctor of internal medicine is in the million-dollar bracket, but quite a few surgeons are."

Surgical techniques and styles change regularly, so who is to say what is and what is not necessary surgery? Surely the patient doesn't know. That is the worrisome province of the medical profession, which is slow to make up its mind, slow to change, and even slower to tell the patient the truth.

Much Too Many Hysterectomies

Take hysterectomies. In 1975, the number of hysterectomies peaked at 725,000 operations a year. The great majority of them, as now, were elective, and ninety percent were done on women with noncancerous conditions. Too often, critics said, the operation was done *instead* of more traditional, less intrusive, medical therapies.

The profession started to rethink the overuse of hysterectomies when estimates of unnecessary operations reached the twenty-five to fifty percent level, putting healthy women at risk of serious complications, even death. The criticism has been working, and the number of such surgeries has been dropping each year.

According to an analysis in the *American Family Physician*, the number of hysterectomies was down to 576,000 a year in 1997.

Does that mean there are no longer unnecessary surgeries on the female uterus? Hardly. *Recent studies indicate that there is still no medical reason to do such an enormous number of hysterectomies, the mainstay of income for many ob/gyn specialists.*

Except in cases such as cancer, it is not usually a life-threatening therapy. The operation is generally done to improve the patient's quality of life. But, critics say, too often the hysterectomy may just be trading one set of distressing symptoms for another. Some permanent sexual dysfunction, for example, is reported as a side effect in up to one-third of hysterectomy patients.

One of the most outspoken critics of unnecessary surgery is Dr. Sidney Wolfe of Public Citizen. "If a doctor immediately says, 'Have a hysterectomy,' shop for a new physician," he suggests. "You need tests to write off all the alternatives."

Southern Women Are Most at Risk

We know that much of the hysterectomy business is unnecessary and that its incidence is influenced by many factors. According to the study of Maine women conducted by the Harvard Medical School, the more educated a woman is and the higher her socioeconomic class, the less chance she will undergo a hysterectomy.

Geography also seems to be factor. If physicians followed solid guidelines on hysterectomy, it would make no difference where patients lived and where doctors practiced. But that's not the case. In the southern states, physicians do the most hysterectomies, at the rate of 83 for every 10,000 women. But in the North, there's almost half as many hysterectomies—48 per 100,000.

Dr. Nina Bickell surveyed 140 North Carolina gynecologists in a study that seemed to confirm a common belief that male doctors did more more hysterectomies than female physicians. But when she corrected for age, the gender gap disappeared. It seems younger gynecologists, which includes more women doctors, do less hysterectomies, which is a hopeful sign.

She also found that patients play a part in unnecessary surgery. When they voiced objections to a hysterectomy for such conditions as painful fibroids, doctors tended to change their opinion that the operation was necessary.

The study of Maine women did show that "appropriate" hysterectomies were effective in relieving the common symptoms of fibroid tumors of the uterus (lieomyomas that are noncancerous and can be as large as a grapefruit), abnormal bleeding, and chronic pelvic pain. But it also indicated that many of these symptoms were also helped by medical treatment, including antihormonal drugs.

The question is: When is hysterectomy necessary and when is it not?

Over Forty Percent Doubtful Surgery

A major study to answer that daunting question was carried out by a group of researchers connected with Rand and the Universities of Michigan and UCLA, done for the Health Maintenance Organization Quality of Care Consortium, and reported in *JAMA*. They studied 5,126 patients whose median age was forty-four. Seventy-five percent were married and 88 percent had children.

The result? Fifty-eight percent of the operations were considered "appropriate," 25 percent were classified as "uncertain," and 16 percent were labeled "inappropriate," or unnecessary. If we extrapolate that to all 576,000 hysterectomies done in America each year, 92,000 women, most of child-bearing age, unnecessarily submitted themselves to the knife. In addition, a quarter of the total hysterectomies were doubtful, leaving the decision of surgical necessity up in the air for another 144,000 women.

In total, 236,000 women were put at risk without surgical certainty.

Unnecessary C-sections

If hysterectomies win the silver medal in the surgical excess competition, then the nearly one-million-a-year cesarean surgeries merit the gold. But why, one might ask, are there so many women electing, or being persuaded by doctors, to have their children come into this world through the abdomen instead of the vagina?

The American Hospital Association has some answers, as do other critics. The reasons seem to be:

- To save the mother or the child in cases of a prolapsed umbilical cord, cases of active genital herpes, problems with the size of the child's head in relation to the mother's pelvis, or a problem with the placenta.
- Cesarean births are sometimes more convenient for doctors who don't want to wait out a long labor.
- Some women patients prefer a C-section to avoid the pain of vaginal birth.
- Some patients believe the C-section will lessen damage to their figures.
- Many doctors believe the operation is part of defensive medicine against malpractice—that it lessens delivery problems stemming from normal vaginal birth.
- Physicians make more money doing a C-section than a regular delivery.

So are many of the 920,000 C-sections unnecessary? Absolutely. In fact, a great many are. Some have even referred to the modern rash of cesareans as a "surgical epi-demic." Calling on understatement, the American College of Obstetricians and Gynecologists admits that C-sections "are more common than they should be." An actual estimate, made by the Centers for Disease Control, says that 349,000 of the cesarean surgeries were unnecessary.

This is a serious situation. The operation is major surgery, and when inappropriate, carries two to four times greater risk to the mother than normal vaginal birth.

Public Citizen, which puts out a regular report on the rate of C-sections, believes the surgery is done almost twice as often as medically indicated, at a cost of an extra $1.3 billion and unnecessary pain and injury.

Like hysterectomy, the rate of C-sections varies geo-graphically, which of course makes no medical sense. The highest rates are in the South and at large for-profit hospitals, where a buck is overappreciated. The worst states are Arkansas, Louisiana, Mississippi, Texas, Alabama, Kentucky, and also Washington, D.C. A northern offender is New Jersey, which, like the southern states, has a C-section rate of over 24 percent. The lowest rate is in Colorado (16 percent), followed by Alaska, Minnesota, and Wisconsin.

Although C-sections are ostensibly done by doctors to reduce the risk of malpractice, they can also result in stimulating malpractice suits from injured women, as in our earlier anecdote.

Unnecessary Back Surgery

Unnecessary surgery waxes and wanes. First one operation, like tonsillectomy, is in fashion, then another, like C-sections. The most recent "in" technique is "back surgery."

The problem of low back pain is one that perplexes the medical establishment, which has yet to find an answer. Up to ninety percent of adults experience it at some time of their lives, what some flippantly say is the price humans pay for walking upright on two feet.

Back pain is the most frequent reason for visits to orthopedic surgeons and neurosurgeons and the second leading reason for all physician visits. Its cost, in health treatments and lost time, comes to $50 billion a year. Little wonder that it has captured the attention of surgeons, even though the U.S. Institute of Medicine has concluded that "surgery for chronic back pain is overused and often misused."

A forceful critic of much back surgery is Dr. Richard A. Deyo, professor at the University of Washington School of Medicine. He points out that most low back pain is caused by a simple muscle strain, which over time heals itself. It is *not*, he says, usually caused by herniated disks in the spine, which are the target of most surgeries.

Dr. Deyo estimates that "diskectomy," the name of such surgery, is performed on 300,000 people a year, and is often a wasteful, unnecessary activity. A diskectomy involves cutting through the bony parts of the vertebrae to remove the jellylike substance inside. The reason is that in herniated disks, the substance protrudes, putting pressure on the nerves.

In some cases this operation only causes more harm. Cutting the bone can weaken the back, so a second procedure may be done during the same operation—fusing vertebrae to shore them up, using a graft of bone, often from the pelvis. There has been a hundred percent rise in fusions in the last ten years.

Dr. Deyo, writing in the journal *Spine*, says America is undergoing an unnecessary back surgery epidemic of such proportions that surgeons here perform diskectomies forty percent more often than other Western nations and *five times more often than in England and Scotland*. It also appears that the number of back surgeries relates directly to the number of appropriate surgeons available in the nation according to population.

In the same publication, Dr. Deyo and others also studied hospitalization for back pain and found that from 1979 to 1990, *nonsurgical* hospitalizations decreased dramatically. Meanwhile, admissions for surgery increased substantially, especially in the South. Nationwide, low back operations among people twenty or older increased from 147,500 to 279,000 in that same period.

This rapidly growing field is under attack from several sources, including a federal bureau, the Agency for Health Care Policy Research (AHCPR), which was established nine years ago to study whether commonly accepted medical treatments actually work. By searching out the scientific literature for "outcome studies," they try to advise doctors and the public on the reality of medical therapies.

They studied the surgical treatment for the common complaint of "low back pain," and concluded that most of the operations were unnecessary. In fact, says the agency, the less treatment for these pains, surgical or medical, the better. A report in the *New England Journal of Medicine*, for instance, decried the use of corticosteroids as risky and of little value. The evidence, says the federal agency, shows that regular activity rather than bed rest reduces the chances of developing a chronic condition that leads to surgery.

The back surgeons have complained that in financing such studies, the government is interfering in their business, which is quite true. But as medicine is presently constituted, there is little choice. The profession itself does very little to evaluate its own work, leaving outside groups like Washington to fill the policing void.

Is It Only a Pain in the Neck?

Surgery is unnecessary when the risk is greater than the benefit, *or* when there is no strong evidence that the surgery will benefit most of the people operated on.

Increasingly, this unfortunate equation is being applied to a common surgery called "carotid endarterectomy," which is now performed on some 130,000 Americans each year. The two carotid arteries go from the heart through the neck to the brain, where the blood nourishes the cells that keep us alive and thinking. When either of the carotid arteries is heavily blocked with fatty plaque, physicians believe it increases the chances for a stroke, a major bleeding into the brain that causes paralysis, blindness, loss of speech, and often leads to an early death.

The "endarterectomy" operation was devised to clean out the built-up plaque in the neck arteries in the hope of preventing strokes. The problem of "stenosis," or narrowing of the blood channel through the carotid artery, can be diagnosed by observing the "bruits" or sounds through a stethoscope.

However, there can be bruits without significant blockage. That diagnostic technique can be followed up by an ultrasound scan and a study of the blood flow in the artery. If there appears to be a narrowing, the doctor can do an MRI scan or a cerebral angiography to determine the size and location of the blockage.

The major appropriate use of the surgery seems to be when there is severe blockage and/or when the patient has already had a "transient ischemic attack" (TIA), in which there is a brain disturbance caused by a temporary deficiency in the brain's blood supply.

Small pieces of fatty material and calcium on the wall of the artery break off and block the blood flow to the brain. The attack generally lasts from two minutes to a half hour and can cause weakness or paralysis on one side of the body, partial loss of hearing and vision, slurred speech, and other problems. But unlike stroke, they are temporary and reversible.

The common carotid endarterectomy surgery is designed to prevent a full-fledged stroke. But is it often overused and unnecessary, especially when there is insufficient diagnosis?

Apparently yes, to a fault.

It seems that enthusiastic (or greedy) surgeons often delve into the artery without proof that the operation is necessary and will help. A study done by the Rand Corporation along with the Department of Medicine and Public Health of UCLA indicates that too many of these operations are unnecessary, even dangerous.

The team studied 1,302 random cases of Medicare patients who had the operation in three geographic areas, and found that "in all three sites a substantial proportion of use was inappropriate." Factors that would make the operation sound include having one or more TIAs, and an observable stenosis or narrowing of the blood channel in the artery that was operated on.

The result? Says the report in the *New England Journal of Medicine:*

"Overall, thirty-two percent of the carotid endarterectomies were performed for inappropriate reasons." They decided that too many operations were done when the stenosis was minimal or there had been no TIAs. Another reason for the surgery being "inappropriate" was that many of the older patients were at high risk for surgery.

There was also considerable postoperative danger. Forty-four patients, or 3.4 percent, died within thirty days of surgery. Over six percent of the patients developed a stroke during or shortly after the surgery. An additional 1.8 percent of the patients—about twenty-four cases—suffered heart attacks.

Their conclusion: "In the absence of solid clinical evidence that the procedure reduces the risk of stroke, and because of the high rate of complications we observed, the use of this procedure should be curtailed and perhaps limited to surgeons and hospitals performing few inappropriate procedures, with acceptable rates of complications."

Another study financed by the National Institute of Neurological Disorders and Stroke found that when not indicated the operation can cause the very strokes it was supposed to prevent. They state that the operation is beneficial when at least 70 percent of the arteries were blocked. However, if the blockage was less than fifty percent, the operation was more dangerous than the potential stroke.

Unnecessary Bypass Operations

Coronary artery bypass operations have had a better record than the neck artery surgery. Earlier studies of the heart operation—in 1979, 1980, and 1982—also showed some evidence of surgical mayhem. Fourteen percent of the surgeries were "inappropriate" or unnecessary, defined as "performing the procedure under circumstances where the medical risk exceeded the medical benefits." The fourteen percent was high, but much less than the carotid surgical extravagance. But the unnecessary rate for bypass operations has now been reduced considerably by new techniques and better choices by patients.

A team from Rand, Harvard School of Public Health, UCLA School of Medicine, and the University of Michigan, studied 1,338 patients who had bypass graft surgery in New York State. They concluded that only 2.4 percent—or some twenty-two patients—were operated on unnecessarily. Auditors concluded that an additional seven percent of the cases were "uncertain"—they weren't sure if the operation was needed or not. Two percent died and seventeen percent did have some complications, the unfortunate by-product of such serious surgeries.

The authors were pleased with the low unnecessary surgery rate, pointing out that patients with less severe heart disease are now being treated medically. The low rate of unnecessary surgery, they concluded, was greatly achieved by the oversight and feedback of the Cardiac Advisory Committee and the Department of Health of New York State, which played a major role in improving the situation.

Solutions to the Surgical Crisis

Overall, how many patients undergo unnecessary operations each year in all forms of surgery?

No one really knows, but it is surely more than a million, perhaps several million. What can stem the tide? Consider the following solutions:

I. Some way should be found to reduce the surgeon's vested financial interest in cutting a patient. At Yale–New Haven Hospital, for example, the surgeons are faculty members on a salary.

II. Surgeons must be encouraged to do more thorough diagnoses before they operate. There is excellent technology for that, much of which is often overlooked. The state medical societies, or the state departments of health, should prepare a diagnostic checklist for specific ailments, which surgeons and patients should study before surgery is attempted.

III. We need to stop the present professional system of *one* surgeon making the decision to cut or not to cut. This is a jealously guarded prerogative of the profession, but one that is an anachronism in today's world and must be eliminated. We often hear the phrase: "Get a second opinion." But few patients, and even fewer surgeons, do.

That must now become a formal requirement for all surgery, enforced by hospitals, or by the states themselves. *Before any patient is placed on the operating table in America, there should be a second concurring opinion signed by another surgeon.* That is a radical departure in professional tradition, but one that is necessary if we are to drastically cut down the scourge of unnecessary surgery.

IV. Rather than wait for a complaint before checking the surgical activity of a doctor, hospitals should conduct routine audits of all surgeries done in their hospital. Afterward, they should announce to the staff which operations they believe were necessary and which were not. The peer pressure of such action will surely reduce the number of abusive operations that might only serve to make the doctor richer.

Just as one surgical operation—like tonsillectomy—is shot down by intelligent criticism, another, like C-section, rises to take its place in the inventory of often unnecessary surgeries. It is now up to the profession—or if forced, the states—to stop the excess cutting stimulated by either greed, medical fashion, or ignorance. That is the only way to protect the unknowing patient public.

Chapter VI

The Making of a
Modern Doctor

Coddling the Medical School Student:
Easy In, Easy Through

Why all this talk about medical incompetence and the enormous difference in the level of quality care from doctor to doctor?

Don't the medical schools take in the best qualified college graduates to train as doctors?

Aren't the medical colleges turning out well-educated, competent physicians?

Don't the schools weed out the worst of the would-be physicians?

What about the licensing of doctors? Isn't that a strict procedure that makes sure the incompetents among medical school graduates never get to practice on you?

Don't the states require physicians to continue their education and keep up?

Unfortunately, the answer to all these questions—in the main—is no.

The reality is that the rumored high standards of training and licensing of doctors in America is patently false. In fact, in no profession are the standards as lax and are so few weeded out in the process of the "making of a doctor."

Much of the disparity from doctor to doctor—which studies indicate exists—starts with the general permissiveness in selection and training, a kind of "gentleman's agreement" for which patients eventually suffer.

Death of the Traditional Doctor

When we think of the traditional physician, the Dr. Marcus Welby so sympathetically played on television by Robert Young, what comes to mind is the image of a male of Anglo or European background, gentile or Jewish (with a disproportionate number of Jews, as in "my son, the doctor"). They were chosen for their skill in science, both in grades and scores on the MCAT, the Medical College Aptitude Test.

Their success, in the 1950s through the 1980s, was heralded throughout the world. Surely, the praise was often excessive, but no one doubted that in the complex specialties and subspecialties of heart transplants, dialysis of kidney patients, cancer treatment, orthopedic repair, and cardiac bypasses, American medicine was the toast of the world. Patients came to our institutions, from the Mayo Clinic to Memorial Sloan-Kettering Cancer Center in New York, from around the world—as they still do.

So what has changed?

Virtually everything. We can't see it, but the selection of students has been altered *dramatically*, as has the licensing process, one which is basically flawed anyway.

First, the selection of medical students is no longer a search for the most scientifically inclined. Instead, a large portion of new medical students are chosen on the basis of "affirmative action," making social goals more important than medical ones.

Let's take a look at the present class of medical students as described in a profile published by the American Association of Medical Colleges. Of the 16,165 entering students: the makeup is as follows, first by gender:

- Males, 9,170 (57 percent).
- Women, 6,995 (43 percent). In nineteen medical schools, women made up a majority of the places.

In terms of race and ethnic group, the makeup is:

- Whites, 10,504 (65 percent).
- Minorities, including African-Americans, Hispanic, native Indians, Asians, and Pacific Islanders, 5,531, or 35 percent. (The numbers don't add up exactly because of 130 foreign students.)

Perhaps the most startling statistic is that Anglo and European-ethnic males, once the strong mainstay of the profession, with perhaps 90 percent of all doctors, now represent only 38 percent of the new students, or a little more than one-third the slots!

So what? one might ask.

Since all were surely chosen on their skills and aptitude, what difference does it make what gender, what race, and what ethnic background medical students are?

Unfortunately, it makes a great deal of difference, if only because a large proportion of medical school students are not chosen for their skills or intelligence, but because of their gender, or their race and ethnic background.

Is that possible? Quite. In fact, in the case of women, for example, the AAMC frankly states:

"For the last three years, equivalent proportions of women and men have been accepted [into medical schools] despite the tendency of women to score lower than men on most parts of the Medical College Admission Test and to have a slightly lower science GPA [Grade Point Average.]"

How much lower do women score in the physical science exam, the mainstay of doctor knowledge?

Considerably. *In the MCAT physical science test, men scored 14 percent higher than the women who were admitted into medical college. In the biological science test, men scored 10 percent higher.* Yet both sexes were admitted in the same proportion as those who applied—57 to 43 percent. In laymen's terms, the MCAT scores represent a mark of 90 for men and approximately 75 for women, the difference between an A and a C. Yet, higher-scoring men are rejected and their places taken by lower-scoring women.

The difference between the present medical school class and those of the past is also shown in the number of "minority" students who are often admitted with relatively low scores in place of higher-scoring nonminority applicants.

A study by the Association of American Medical Colleges called "Minority Students in Medical Education" speaks of them as a new category of doctors—"URM," or "underrepresented." The implication is that the medical profession should have the same proportion of racial, gender, and ethnic groups as Americans in general, regardless of their qualifications. This is an illogical, destructive concept in such a vital, lifesaving profession.

Even though the new selection system endangers medical quality, the URM theory is vigorously enforced in the medical schools. While the number of white male students drops each year, and the size of the entering student body remains constant at approximately 16,000, the number of women and minority students rises continually. African-American medical school enrollments have gone up by 26 percent; Native American medical students by 81 percent; and Mexican-Americans by 60 percent.

Is this happening because of increased superiority of minority students?

No. The unfortunate reality is that the minority doctors-to-be are not only admitted with lower college grades, but with a thirty percent comparative deficiency on the MCAT physical science test—too low to guarantee that they can become effective physicians.

Did these minority students come from poor families who take the brunt of lowered opportunities? Hardly. An AAMC report shows that their annual family income was $61,952, which puts them in the upper strata of America, hardly the profile of inner-city youngsters.

Doctors Defending Doctors

To defend themselves, deans of medical colleges say that there are factors other than science that can determine a doctor's quality, such as how well a student interviews, his or her community service, philosophy of life, extracurricular activities, compassion, etc., all parts of the equation of who should be our doctors.

This theory that science is not all-important mirrors the horrible medicine of the nineteenth century, when there was little knowledge and doctors were compassionate, even to the point of making house calls at all hours of the night, and sitting by the bedside as the patient slowly died.

Of course, there is no proof that women or minorities selected for medical training are any more compassionate than prior candidates. One dean stated that females, for example, are given some preference as credit for their "life experiences" and how well they interview, vague, subjective concepts that have no objective meaning.

If a young woman or minority doctor has been admitted into medical school in place of a more scientifically qualified person, does the patient (male or female) really care that the doctor played the tuba in high school, or even "interviewed well," as they say?

As we have seen over the past half century, science has been the *sole* factor that has made modern medicine meaningful. In fact, the eminent medical historian, Arthur K. Shapiro, former clinical professor at Mt. Sinai, has explained, as we've seen, that until the medical scientific revolution truly began in World War II, doctors probably destroyed more lives than they saved.

The revolution that created higher standards of medicine began with the Flexner Report of 1910, authored by Thomas Flexner, a former high school teacher and son of German-Jewish immigrants. He discovered that most medical schools were diploma mills, unscientific to a fault, where often ignorant mentors taught their biases—including "bleeding" for many ailments and "suction cups" for pneumonia—to willing apprentices improperly schooled even in the few things we did know at the time.

As a result of his study, state legislatures closed most of the medical schools and required that the remaining ones (and new ones) become affiliated with universities, creating the present system.

The rationale for now choosing students less capable in science is explained as an attempt at "gender, racial, and ethnic" balance, ostensibly to make up for supposed prior discrimination.

But simply put, that claim of "prior discrimination" against women, for instance, is not true. For some time there has been absolutely no discrimination against women seeking to become doctors. In 1960, for instance, 7 percent of all applicants to medical school were women. And acceptances? The very same 7 percent. There was no discrimination. What was missing was the *desire* among women to become physicians, one which is very much changed today.

But what if there were no affirmative action? What would the present class at medical schools look like? Would the 43 percent of new medical students still be female if the only objective measure of scientific knowledge—the MCAT test—was used as the criterion? Hardly. Judging from the scores published by the American Association of Medical Colleges, that 43 percent would probably drop below 20 percent.

In the case of minorities, the current enrollment, which is between 15 and 20 percent nationwide, would probably shrink by two-thirds.

Do any of the affirmative action doctors see their role differently than other medical school graduates? Apparently they do.

Once in actual practice, for instance, women seem to choose a different path from the men. In surgery, only one in twenty-two female doctors choose that difficult specialty, for example. Though 61 percent of the new residents in pediatrics are women, only eight female doctors are training for pediatric surgery in the entire nation. Only seven women are training in colon and rectal surgery.

Heart surgery produces similar disheartening statistics. Today, a half-million coronary bypass operations are performed each year. There are now 2,293 male cardiac surgeons and only 45 women.

But surely that's an historic accident based on an era when there were few female doctors. Wrong. A study of all six years of surgical residency shows that only fourteen women are in training in cardiac surgery in the nation. Who will do the expected one million life-extending coronary bypass operations in years to come?

Permanent Disparity in Scores

But surely, skeptics might ask, won't the medical school students less equipped in science make up for their poorer scores once they are trained? Doesn't the relative deficiency in the MCAT test scores disappear after they have studied for two years in the basic medical sciences?

Apparently not. In fact, the spread stays the same or even increases, confirming the original disparity.

Beth Dawson, a professor at Southern Illinois University School of Medicine, has studied the scientific test performance from the point of view of the gender, race, and ethnicity of medical students, and reported her findings in *JAMA*. Her results showed that on Step One of the medical licensing test, which is taken midway through medical school and measures scientific knowledge, white males had the highest scores, women in general scored considerably lower, while the minority students performed even worse.

Dr. Dawson's co-author, Dr. Thomas Bowles of the National Board of Medical Examiners, noted: "What you're seeing is a reflection of affirmative action programs taken on by medical schools. This is a healthy mission and it's going to involve some trade-off along the way."

Dr. Bowles may be sanguine about the "trade-offs" that come from choosing inferior students in the name of a social—not medical—mission. But that view may not be shared by a patient whose life may depend on the scientific skill of the physician searching out the right chemotherapy mix for breast cancer or doing a coronary bypass operation.

Beth Dawson's longitudinal study covered the first part of what is now the three-part U.S. Medical Licensing Exam (USMLE). Passing that three-step examination satisfies the written requirements for being licensed as a doctor in all fifty states of the union, as well as in Canada.

The passing grade, from 0 to 100, is 75. The white male students—the old stereotypical American physicians—scored the highest, with 90 percent passing. Next were the Asian males, 87 percent of whom passed. After that were the women in general, 79 percent of whom passed. Only 66 percent of the Hispanic students passed, as did 54 percent of the black males. The lowest percentage was achieved by black women, only 44 percent of whom passed the two-year science exam.

The Actual Scores Are Even Lower

But the results for all the medical students—males, females, and minorities—are even worse than one might imagine. We are all familiar with what a grade of 75 usually means: answering three-fourths of the questions correctly, a mediocre performance that invites both hope and ridicule. But the 75 grade on the USMLE is lower than the conventional C grade. It is closer to what we normally associate with an F.

"The passing grade on the USMLE," Dr. Bowles explains, "means that the student has correctly answered between fifty-five and sixty percent of the questions."

Should a doctor who has failed to help a patient then explain that he passed his licensing exam, but didn't answer almost half the medical science questions, one of which involves the problem he was now facing?

Is the test at fault, as some inevitably claim?

Professor Dawson says absolutely not. In fact, the scores were "corrected" to compensate for the lower admissions criteria of women and minorities. Otherwise the spread in the scores would be even larger.

"There's certainly no evidence that the test is biased with respect to minorities," she has stated. "I wouldn't say it's biased with respect to women."

Dr. Bowles has been quoted as stating that knowledge of science is not all that it takes to become a good doctor. However, he admits that it is a starting point. "It's very hard to be a good doctor unless you are knowledgeable."

Amen. Every patient would agree.

Truly Permissive Med Schools

But surely, one would assume that there's a failproof method to compensate for these low scores. Wouldn't the poorer medical students flunk out of medical college before the end of four years? Can the medical establishment afford to allow them to practice on live patients—meaning you and me?

Apparently so. Incompetence is well-tolerated in the medical establishment. Very few students flunk out of medical school for academic reasons.

In fact, of the 16,289 students in a recent fourth-year graduating class, only *fifty-one* would-be doctors, or *one-third of one percent*, were dismissed for academic reasons, the lowest failure rate of any institution from high school up. Another study, this one conducted by the AMA, showed that of 67,000 medical students in all 126 medical schools, only 207—or the same one-third of one percent of students—were dismissed for academic reasons.

"Almost no one flunks out for academic failure," confirms the dean for admissions at the Yale School of Medicine, who then adds the party line: "We carefully select our people so that they will succeed."

That self-protective comment is designed to thwart criticism of their policy of bias against higher-skilled male students in favor of lower-scoring women and minorities. The false theory also protects those among the white and Asian male students who perform poorly as well. Med school's laxity is absolutely unbiased.

By now one would hope that the licensing exam would catch the incompetent young physicians—of whatever gender or race—even if the school lets them graduate for social and political reasons.

Unfortunately, it will not.

On its *surface*, the three-step licensing test sounds impressive:

Step One: At the end of the second year, the students take the United States Medical Licensing Exam (USMLE) on their command of biomedical knowledge. The exam includes 720 items administered over two days. (To help the students pass, a booklet "containing the detailed content outline and sample items" is published each year, a kind of academic pony.)

How did they do? Of the 16,800 students who took the Step One test in June 1996, 93 percent passed the first time. Those who failed, retook it in October and 57 percent of them passed. Overall, 88 percent of all would-be doctors passed in that year.

Step Two: This exam, given in the fourth year of medical school, tests whether students can apply their scientific knowledge in a clinical setting. It is an attempt to simulate the practice of medicine, but under supervision, such as received by an intern in a hospital. The total passing rate was 90 percent, including repeaters.

Step Three: This exam is given at the end of the first postgraduate year, when the new doctor finishes his internship. As the USMLE states, "Step Three assesses whether an examinee can apply the medical knowledge and understanding of biomedical and clinical science considered essential for the unsupervised practice of medicine, with emphasis on patient management in ambulatory setting." More simply said, it's a test of how well the doctor will able to deliver medical care on his own once he is in practice.

On this exam, 95 percent of the students passed on the first try. In all, it seems that about 93 percent of students passed all three tests on the first try, and that 7 percent, or about a thousand would-be doctors, failed.

Does this mean that they have been rejected as future physicians? No. They merely take the test again. This time about sixty percent pass.

What about the remainder of the students? Are they doomed to never administer—even if inaccurately—to patients?

Hardly. Until 1992, students could take the licensing exam only three times, much like the bar exam. Three strikes and you were out. But that year, the two licensing boards combined and recommended to the states that med students be allowed to take the new USMLE test up to *six* times.

The profession has now decided to become even more permissive in protecting doctors and punishing patients. Having filled the student roster with a large group of unlikely candidates, and having rejected the more competent for the less competent, there is still another touch of medical permissiveness, if not insanity, to face up to.

Many state licensing boards have since passed legislation *permitting students to take the USMLE an unlimited number of times, possibly forever, until they get it right.* That is, the test, if not the practice of medicine.

In the final analysis, three years after graduation, more than 99 percent of all students will have passed the examination that will license them in all fifty states of the nation. Protection for the public against incompetent and semieducated doctors is not part of the current medical equation.

The Failure of Foreign Medical Schools

What about doctors trained elsewhere? How do they do on the USMLE?

If medical training in America is lax, it is much worse in the undeveloped nations of the world. Graduates of foreign medical schools who want to practice in the United States and Canada must take a test administered by the Educational Commission for Foreign Medical Graduates (ECFMG).

Their results are lower than that of American graduates. In 1996, 16,869 graduates of foreign schools took the Step One test, and only 55 percent passed the first time. The total for Step Three was higher, a total of 69 percent. In all, in 1996, some 7,000 graduates of foreign schools were licensed to practice in America in addition to the 16,000 homegrown doctors.

In With the Old . . .

Once he has his license, is there anything else that a doctor *must* do to maintain his standing in the profession and with the state. Surely, there must be rules that require them to keep up with new advances. Surely, they are required to read journals. Surely, they must attend classes periodically at the local medical school to maintain their licenses. Surely, they must take periodic examinations to prove they still know what they're doing.

Wrong again. The autonomous American doctor who may have barely scraped through medical college and barely passed the insufficient USMLE licensing exam is on his own, determining his own variant of medicine. Unless he has misbehaved, he generally will have no contact with the state licensing authority that allows him to practice medicine and surgery. Like a Supreme Court justice, he's in for life—no matter how much modern medicine may be passing him by.

In Connecticut, for example, there once *was* a proviso that required doctors to complete sixty hours of continuing education a year. But that was waived in the 1980s. Now a Connecticut doctor can legally maintain his license and practice as he sees fit with no intrusion by the state. All he needs to do is send in his $450 yearly fee.

The Federation of State Medical Boards in Texas has developed a "Special Purpose Exam" (or SPEX) that will tell the state if doctors are keeping up. The six-hour test, as a spokesman commented, "is more current, but not as intense as the original license exam."

Connecticut ostensibly has an agreement with the FSMB to give the exam, but a state spokesman pointed out that it is not used except if a doctor is in trouble or must legally be recertified after leaving and returning to the state. Otherwise, the $450 yearly payment for the doctor's medical license is more important than whether he or she still knows their business—or ever did.

In New York and New Jersey, centers of intense medical practice, nothing is required of doctors after licensure except to pay their fee. There is no requirement for continuing education and no reexam after a number of years. Caveat emptor. Patient beware.

In fact, the FSMB explains that *no* state requires that doctors take the SPEX exam to show they have maintained their knowledge. It is used only in cases of special discipline, as the name implies.

The Tragic Lack of Continuing Education

The lack of continuing education is a drain on the profession, making quality care almost impossible in the hands of the average doctor. An avalanche of new information pours out of the medical journals, many of which go unread by physicians. *So dire is that situation that the American Medical Association is now offering Continuing Medical Education credits to doctors just for reading the profession's basic journal,* JAMA.

The program, which began in November 1997, asks doctors to read three of the designated eight articles in each issue, answer questions about them, and fax their responses to the AMA. Like students in freshman college classes, the doctors are asked whether they agree or disagree with questions like, "I plan to seek more information on this topic," or "I plan to discuss this information with colleagues." The hope, says the AMA, is that physicians will use "this information to change their medical practices for the better."

The editors of *JAMA* add the most damaging statement on the inadequacy of the intellect and learning habits of American doctors. "Unfortunately, as the methods and clinical utility of articles published in primary-source, peer-reviewed medical journals continue to improve, fewer physicians are taking the time to read these journals. . . ."

There is something almost pitiful in having to bribe physicians into reading medical journals, something that could improve their practice and save lives, something that should be as automatic with them as eating and walking. But that is the nature of the ignorance that often permeates the field, especially in knowledge of new research that could be lifesaving.

JAMA offers an example of this ignorance in a recent article entitled, "Bridging the Gap Between Research and Practice: The Role of Continuing Medical Education." The authors cite a study, "Adverse Outcomes of the Underuse of (Beta-) Blockers in Elderly Survivors of Acute Myocardial Infarction." The study focused on Medicare patients in New Jersey who had heart attacks, and found that only 23 percent of the eligible patients had been given beta-blockers by their doctors.

On follow-up, it turned out that those few who had received the treatment had a 43 percent lower death rate and 23 percent less hospitalization than those who had not received beta-blockers. Similar studies on younger patients showed the same result. This was all confirmation of research that has been published *over the last fifteen years*, including one study of 35,000 patients.

Research Is Ignored by Doctors

But apparently, the research fell on deaf physician ears—and blind eyes—that apparently do not hear or read, or do not care about continuing medical education. Too often, doctors are stuck in the therapeutic parameters they learned in medical school.

The authors of this *JAMA* piece demonstrate the slow learning habits of many of their colleagues. The National Registry of Myocardial Infarction cataloguing the 240,989 heart patients from 1990 to 1993, for instance, explained that only 36 to 42 percent of them received beta-blocker therapy, what the authors called "underusage." Even cardiologists used the proven therapy only 48 percent of the time.

Even when they do learn, physicians often backslide. "There is some evidence," say the *JAMA* piece authors, "that practice change is not sustained after a particular stimulus to intervention is withdrawn, suggesting that ongoing reinforcement may be needed."

One would think he was talking to recalcitrant children rather than physicians!

New Laxity in Board Certification

In the often insufficient education of doctors, one important hurdle, as we've seen, is getting one's "boards." It's not legally necessary, but according to the American Board of Medical Specialties in Evanston, Illinois, some two-thirds of all physicians are board certified, which still leaves some 225,000 doctors without that imprimatur.

There are twenty-six specialty boards, which give out diplomas in thirty-six specialties and seventy-three sub-specialties. The problem is that even the specialty boards are becoming more lax—following the lead of permissive medical colleges.

Most boards have a time period in which doctors may apply after finishing their hospital residencies, or, in the case of subspecialties, their extended hospital fellowships. The American Board of Internal Medicine, for example, *used* to allow candidates to take the certification exam four times over a period of six years if they failed the first time.

But apparently someone found that too taxing, and now—since July 1, 1996—candidates can take the test ad infinitum, an unlimited number of times, until they are gray-of-beard. Ten other specialty boards have that same permissive attitude, which does not serve the patient well. After a while even the poorest doctors can get the hang of a difficult test.

Some Good News: Two Trends in Medical Education

There are perhaps two positive new trends in medical education. Pioneered at Harvard and other medical schools, students are being introduced to live patients from the beginning of their education. Rather than wait until the third "clinical" year, when some critics believe the students have already been "dehumanized" by the concentration on science, however necessary, freshmen are introduced to the hospital care system early on.

That's a wise policy. *Without lessening the importance of concentrated science training, all schools should provide for some patient contact in the first year.*

The second new trend, just in its infancy, is a program that takes the student, at various points in his education, *out of the hospital*, a setting where he sees only the sickest of patients. He is periodically rotated through regular physicians' offices, where he sees patients at all stages of illness and gets a truer sample of the type of medical practice he will probably enter. He can even experience the horrendous effects that HMOs are placing on the actual practice of medicine.

Now the Bad News: Two Other Trends

There are, however, two new and even larger trends in medicine that could turn out to be almost as devastating as the flagrant use of affirmative action in selecting new doctors. One is the claim that there are now too many doctors, and that we have to cut back on the number of physicians by twenty percent!

That is the recommendation of the Pew Health Professions Commission, which also wants to close twenty percent of the medical schools to eleviate the "oversupply" of doctors. Simultaneously, they want to reduce the number of "residency" postgraduate slots in hospitals from the current 24,000 to 15,400.

"Oversupply" of doctors is news to many patients, who must wait weeks for an appointment with a good specialist and who find that there are seldom residents around to help them in the hospital. Also, the supposed oversupply—if it existed—should create more competition and push down the price of medicine. That hasn't happened, except through the crass commercialism of the HMO business, which has given the doctors an ultimatum to save money and, in their role as insurance people, allowed themselves, in effect, to practice medicine without a license.

In fact, the Pew Commission uses the HMO devastation as one of the reasons why we should graduate fewer doctors. Speaking of an "emerging health system" dominated by managed care organizations, they say that medical schools must accommodate themselves. In reality, the HMOs should do the adapting.

The academic community is up in arms at the suggestion, as they should be. University hospitals have been the backbone of quality care, and closing twenty-five or more of them will be devastating to any hope of ever achieving the elusive goal of *uniformly* good medicine. "These institutions are tremendously important in their communities," warns Dr. William Jacott, a member of the AMA board of trustees, "and the impact of closing would go far beyond the faculty, to hit the students in the pipeline, the ongoing research, and the staffs that depend on the facilities. . . ."

The Pew people have also failed to study demographic trends. Everyone in the profession knows that the aged on Medicare require two to three times as much medical care as younger people. By the year 2008—less than ten years from now—the baby boomers will start on Medicare, and they will strain, perhaps beyond our imagination, the institutions of medicine. Empty hospitals may start to fill up, and the load on doctors will skyrocket. With the graying of America, this is hardly the time to close twenty percent of our medical schools or train fewer doctors.

But so insistent is Washington to follow the misguided recommendations of the Pew Commission that they have offered the 42 teaching hospitals in the New York area $400 million of taxpayer money to cut back their production of physicians over the next six years by admitting fewer doctors to their residency programs!

Reducing the number of postgraduate medical residents is a ludicrous idea. Attending doctors are so busy in lucrative private practices that they leave too much of specialty care in hospitals to overworked residents whose ranks are thin.

Recently, New York University Medical Center was fined $16,000 by the state because their surgical residents worked more than the legal maximum of eighty hours a week—up to 130 hours, or almost nineteen hours a day. An investigation of twelve leading New York hospitals showed that all of them were breaking the law by overworking the thin line of residents. Yet the Pew Commission wants to cut their ranks by twenty percent!

"It strikes me as ironic that, at a time when baby boomers are about to retire and the needs of an aging population are going to markedly increase demands on the health care system, we are cutting back on graduate medical education slots," writes Dr. Lee Balablan to *JAMA*. "The idea that Medicare is paying hospitals not to train residents is ludicrous. Through research, we have increased the knowledge base and specialization of medicine, which increases the need for specialists."

Another ridiculous scheme, this one also orchestrated by the Department of Health and Human Services, is eroding the number of specialists and placing increased emphasis on the production of "primary care" doctors. This is done by changing the allocation of monies to medical schools, especially through government control of some $7 billion in Medicare subsidies. In the urology specialty, for instance, the government has just reduced the number of residency spots available, and put their money into the creation of more primary doctors. Their goal is reportedly to increase the number of graduates in primary care to equal the *combined* number of specialists.

That makes no medical sense. As millions of prostate sufferers will (or should) tell you, any patient who leaves the treatment of that condition to a nonspecialist is a fool. The same is true of anyone with a heart condition, cancer, arthritis, colonitis, diabetes, or any chronic or acute condition that can be either crippling or life-threatening.

"Primary care" looks good on paper, but patients— eventually—learn the hard way that there is too much new medical knowledge for primary doctors to absorb for them to be able to treat complicated illnesses. Once diagnosed by a primary screener, every *intelligent* patient should head for a recognized specialist for his care. (If his HMO will let him!)

Solutions to the Medical Training Crisis

We have outlined a lax system of professional enrollment, training, licensure, and lifetime education, with almost no safeguards in which inferior and incompetent doctors—of whom there are many—will be blocked from practicing on his fellow man.

Does it have to be that way? Of course not. To change the system and provide for a better educated, better selected, better examined body of physicians, it might be wise for patients, politicians, and physicians to examine this compendium of *six reforms*, my remedy for the creation of better doctors and better medical care:

I. All affirmative action in medical schools should be abolished by law in all fifty states. Nothing is as heinous as using those on whom we depend for life and death to be part of an experiment in social balance.

All evidence indicates that many affirmative action medical students, both women and minorities, are inferior students, in general, and, by extrapolation, inferior doctors. Likewise, eliminating these students, who now take up almost a majority of student slots, will permit the admission of superior students who are being turned away by what is becoming an anti-intellectual profession.

To accomplish this, medical students should be chosen solely by the MCAT test, *without* any interview and any knowledge of the applicants' sex, race, or ethnic background. This is the method used by Stuyvesant High School and the Bronx High School of Science, two schools whose excellence is exemplified by the large number of Westinghouse Science scholarships they win. Whoever passes that screen—white males or black women—should become the doctors of the future.

II. The medical schools must change their self-protective attitude in graduating virtually all students. Instead, the entering class should be ten percent *larger* to allow for the elimination of many more students who do not measure up to a much tougher academic scrutiny. This will change the character of the medical establishment, ensuring that only the best will graduate.

III. The national licensing exam is an academic joke, serving only to reinforce the poor selection and grading of doctors. Its 75 passing grade means that the student has answered only 55 to 60 percent of the questions correctly, which in most exams is an F. The complexity of questions should be kept as it is, but the passing grade should mean that the would-be doctor has correctly answered *at least* 75 percent of the questions. This, like the bar exam, will eliminate the bottom rung of would-be doctors.

That's the very least we deserve as patients. And instead of the medical student being able to take the test an unlimited number of times, the old rule of "three strikes and you're out" should be reinstituted.

IV. The enrollment at medical schools should not be reduced, but instead increased by twenty percent, so that not only will the bottom-scoring ten percent fail to graduate, but another ten percent can be eliminated by a tougher licensing exam, much as the bar examination now functions.

V. The new concentration on primary doctors should be dropped as the patient population ages and becomes sicker. That movement should be replaced by renewed emphasis on the creation of subspecialists who can care for the aging baby boomers coming onto Medicare.

VI. Physicians who fail to maintain a high level of new knowledge through compulsory continuing education should be given two chances to properly "keep up," or have their licenses to practice medicine suspended, then possibly revoked.

Americans deserve the best and the brightest to care for them. And the patient, through his governments at all levels, must insist that truly strict standards apply to his doctor all along the professional path—as a medical student, as a candidate for licensure, and as a practicing physician. Anything less violates the spirit of the Hippocratic Oath and endangers the health of the nation.

Chapter VII
Medical Economics and the American Doctor

Business Before Healing

As he spoke to his patient, the physician was careful not to go near the doorknob of the examination room.

No other signal would be more damaging to his careful business plan of squeezing seven patients secretly, but cordially, into an hour. To handle that volume he had to rush, but he couldn't give the appearance of haste. Or as the article in the professional magazine had tutored him: "You Can Be an Eight-Minute Marcus Welby."

That's no easy accomplishment. But he was being helped by the burgeoning profession of "practice management consultants," who now run the time of doctors, trying constantly to increase their "productivity," generally at the expense of the patient. As that article's advice to the avaricious doctor explained, he had to make every minute count.

"I know an old physician who had this magical way

213

of making five minutes seem like a lifetime in patients' eyes," a practice management consultant in Michigan explained. "The secret, he told me, is to focus on the patient . . . and don't *ever* place your hand on the doorknob of the exam room, while either of you is talking."

It's closer to show business than medicine, but doctors find that racing from one patient to another without letting the patient in on the trick pays off. "You have to act like you have all day," a California doctor adds.

One of the secrets is letting the patient talk out his woes at the beginning of his allotted eight minutes. "How can I help you?" is the opening gambit, followed by a full minute of silence on the doctor's part while the patient talks. This apparently works. A Chicago consultant says that the best listeners have the most patients.

Another consultant adds that it's good to get personal, if only for a few seconds of the compressed medical session. He advises that doctors should make notes on the patient's chart about outside activities or family, then throw in a cordial, if calculated, question about a son, daughter, or wife, or even the patient's golf score.

Show Business Pays Off

Does all this hurry-up make-believe work? Yes, exceptionally well.

And besides, as doctors see it, quick patient turnover is increasingly vital to their pocketbook, which has been greatly challenged by the discounted fees paid by HMOs. The answer to managed care, doctors almost unanimously believe (privately), is less time for the patient in exchange for less money from the insurers. All the doctor has to do is to sacrifice his integrity as a healer, an increasingly common phenomenon.

Can a doctor practice good medicine in eight minutes?

Of course not. Occasionally, he can successfully see a patient in that short time, but this is dangerous medicine. If he faces an obvious cold and is satisfied to prescribe vitamin C and aspirin, a few minutes *may* be sufficient. But a rushed doctor is a sloppy doctor, who might be overlooking bronchitis, influenza, or an incipient pneumonia. Surely under the new pressures (some have always managed their schedules too tightly), there's no time for a real physical examination, real and telling questions by either the patient or the doctor, and true contemplative thought.

"Hurry up" medicine also increases the possibility of error. As the University of California at San Diego reported concerning the large increase in outpatient medication errors since 1983 (which we have already covered), part of the problem was that less time is given to each patient by doctors, mainly because of the HMOs.

Good-bye, Hippocrates

So whatever happened to the Hippocratic Oath? Physicians—except, generally, academic doctors—gave that up as impractical a long time ago. The HMOs and their bargain with the devil has only accelerated the gap between the ideals and the actual practice of medicine, making it even more of a business than a healing profession. And if the truth be known, even before the current crisis doctors were excellent small businessmen, having been educated en masse by practice management consultants.

So why does the doctor shirk his ethical duties? First, some doctors don't want to lose patients, and giving each of them more time would mean he'd have to work even longer hours. Second, losing patients could be financially suicidal if HMOs and Medicare further reduce their present payment schedule, which is probable. And third, and perhaps the most important reason, doctors generally have a fixed—rather high—income in mind which they feel they *must* earn.

Why is that? It's a matter of exaggerated ego, and the need for status and a lifestyle to match it. Doctors have the absolute conviction that their incomes must be *much* higher than those of people as "ordinary" as their patients.

A doctor doesn't expect to earn the obscene amounts handed out by Wall Street, but he is convinced that his status in life demands a net income of between $150,000 and $500,000 (with a handful of million-plus surgeons)— depending on his specialty and where he practices. With that comes the Lexus or Mercedes, second homes, good camps for his children, cash for college without student loans, and a *large* retirement nest egg.

Better at Business than Science

In fact, virtually every study to date has shown that most doctors are deficient in the art and science of quality medical care. However, a study of their business acumen would show the opposite. By and large, doctors are better businessmen than they are physicians.

Part of the blame should be placed in the lap of American patients, who don't seem to mind that they are overpaying doctors. In this country there is a mythology that doctors *deserve* their exaggerated incomes, as if incomes must relate to the importance of their work. Scientists, teachers, professors, do very important work, with much lower incomes.

Besides, other nations, including Britain, Germany, France, and Japan, also have highly developed medical professions, yet doctor incomes in those nations are closer to half that of American doctors.

In fact, in Britain, physicians are not generally called "Doctor," but "Mister." The exaggerated income of American physicians is closely related to the exaggerated status, even reverence, with which they're held in America. This despite their general failure to practice quality medicine.

Keeping up that income level takes much of the mental energy of doctors. Years ago, most patients paid the doctor directly, so the physician could gauge his income accurately. Today, almost all his cash flow comes from third parties—federal or state government, the HMOs, and the indemnity insurance companies.

Payment Codes Are Secret

There is no posted, or explained, payment schedule for the patient to peruse, or any way to negotiate with the doctor. The reason is that the doctor is usually paid by insurance "codes" that are unknown to the patient. The doctor will receive pretty much, within reason, what he writes down on his Medicare and insurance forms about the patient visit, including both the diagnosis and treatment.

As we've pointed out, it is an honor system in an era of professional decline in honor, a disease that seems to have engulfed our entire civilization. Many doctors cheat on these forms by upcoding, as explained earlier. But even the honest ones try desperately to receive the highest possible amount by checking off the highest possible codes, an arcane science of sorts.

"Get the Highest Code You're Entitled To," advises a medical magazine, which goes on to explain the almost byzantine maneuvers that will bring more money into the doctor's bank account, and which could make the difference between that summer at the club or a cruise to Europe, and more.

The article gives the example of a family physician who sees 125 patients a week, closer to four patients an hour than the seven of the would-be Marcus Welby on roller skates.

In the case of a typical office visit, if the doctor checks off Code 92213 instead of 92212, which is only marginally different on a Medicare form, he ends up with $60,000 a year more in his pocket and that much less in the coffers of Uncle Sam— that is, me and you.

Is this knowledge of codes something doctors have to master as well as or better than the side effects of the newest antibiotics? Absolutely, especially since each doctor seems to interpret the insurance codes somewhat differently. And those who best master the system will be the richer ones.

Codes Maketh the Doctor

As an experiment, a family physician in Pennsylvania sent a detailed description of an office visit to several doctors and asked them to code it. The results were uniformly nonuniform.

The case involved a woman in her forties who complained of urinary pain. She had been urinating frequently, going to the bathroom eight times during the day, then getting up to urinate during the night. She was nervous and experiencing chest pains. The patient had no previous urinary problems, and there was no history of heart conditions in her family.

The doctor examined her chest and lungs. Her heart was normal, with no murmur, and the lungs were clear. Her urinary tract showed no abnormalities. The doctor ordered a urinalysis and culture and prescribed a sulfa drug for any possible infection.

Should the code be a 99212 for a "Problem Focused" or simple office visit? A 99213 for more extended treatment, an "Expanded Problem Focused" visit, which would bring him an extra ten dollars? Or perhaps he should check off 99214, a "Detailed" diagnosis and treatment, which would give him even more for the visit?

A panel of three "coding experts" who looked at the case decided that while most doctors would chose 99213 because they believe it is accurate, and don't want to risk an audit from Medicare or the insurance company, the correct answer was the more lucrative 99214.

How did they arrive at that? Simply because (and this is hard to believe) the doctor actually took a "history of present illness," meaning the urinary pain, including its location, severity, duration, and associated signs and symptoms. That gave him the "four checked entries" on the Medicare form necessary for the big 99214.

One would think this was just the minimum practice of medicine, but in the jungle of modern medical economics, one never knows.

In addition, the doctor got two points out of three just for asking about "past, family, and social history." This standard third-year medical school technique would award him the even better paying code of 99215—"Comprehensive" treatment!

The form also lists "a review of systems," fourteen of which are involved, from the cardiovascular to musculoskeletal to respiratory. The doctor qualifies for the basic 99212 even if he reviews *none* of them, which seems impossible unless he's not practicing medicine. If he checks that he examined just *one* of the fourteen, he's already eligible for the higher 99213 category. And if he checks two of the fourteen, he moves into the even loftier 99214 code. This doctor checked off four.

So, this simple visit, in which the doctor practiced the minimum possible for anyone with a conscience, suddenly rewards him with a check from Medicare two stages above the basic, from 99212 up to 99214. To label this method of payment—a sort of bribe to do better than a third-year medical student—as reasonable "medical economics" is to insult the disciplines of medicine and economics and the intelligence of the paying patient.

The whole coding system is ludicrous. One must laugh at the minimum requirements of a 99212 office visit. In that, the doctor is required to check off only one item of "history of present illness" from among eight. He can also (follow this carefully) do *no* reviews of the patient's biological systems, and *no* review of past, family, and social history.

Instead of the proper response, which should be a malpractice suit from the patient, or suspension of the doctor's license by the state, he will instead receive a check from Medicare or an insurance company.

Increasingly, the patient is now a code number to many

doctors, one that can enrich him greatly if he plays the game skillfully.

Is it, as we've already asked, significant to his pocketbook? Apparently so, even more than we have suggested. The same family physician who upgrades his coding from 99212 to 99213, as we've seen, takes in $60,000 more a year. But if he listens to the advice of the coding experts—or by happenstance practices reasonable medicine—he can upgrade that same visit to 99214, adding *$100,000* a year or more to his income! If he should, by accident, practice "Comprehensive" medicine, he could probably make enough to get rid of those pesky HMOs.

By a simple slip of the pen, our haphazard doctor can hit the lottery.

This coding nonsense can and should be curtailed immediately. Doctors should be paid a specific amount for each office visit, no matter what they do for the patient. In some cases, the time spent will be short, in others, considerably longer. Instead of game-playing, the physician should be practicing good medicine, including proper history, diagnosis, and treatment *solely* because he's a doctor and not a coding expert.

It's a Living—A *Very* Good Living

What do doctors make? How high are their incomes and are they coming down or going up?

When managed care took off in the early 1990s, doctors whined extravagantly, convinced that their glory days were over. In the 1980s, doctors' incomes were rising some 10 percent per year and satisfied physicians were sure it would last—unless, of course, America followed the primrose path down to socialized medicine.

We didn't get socialized medicine but in the 1990s, managed care and HMOs took off and doctors complained again, fearful that discounted medicine was not the way to get rich.

For a while they were right. The AMA reported that in

1994, for the first time in recent history, doctor income *dropped* nearly four percent. But doomsday has since been put on hold. A recent study by the AMA covering the full year 1996 shows that doctor income has not only rebounded, but has hit an historic high. That year, the AMA reports, doctor income reached an *average* of some $200,000, with specialists like cardiovascular surgeons taking in an average net of $363,000. At the bottom of the specialty barrel were pediatricians, with incomes of *only* $137,000.

The record $200,000 figure is an increase of $18,000, or almost ten percent, over 1994 and $70,000 or about 50 percent, above 1987 when managed care was first coming into its own.

How did they do it when faced with HMO restrictions, paperwork, and confusion? Basically, by being more "productive" and making better use of insurance codes in their billing. And most important, they have been seeing more patients in less time. That naturally brings in more money even if it diminishes the chance to heal.

A closer look at the varied incomes of various types of doctors is best provided by *Medical Economics*, which does a yearly survey. Their figures are in median (half of doctors earned more and half less) numbers. The latest figures also cover the full year of 1996, but we can assume that they are some 10 percent higher today.

The figures show that the typical doctor in America, including those who practice in low-paying rural areas, had a *median* gross income of $274,000 and a net of $160,740. The rise over the previous year was a reasonable 4.7 percent, considerably more than the inflation rate. Naturally, the specialists earned even more than the "primary" doctors.

Among the biggest gainers were cardiologists, whose median net rose to $240,780, heart surgeons, whose net jumped eleven percent to $278,000 (with a gross of $427,000), and anesthesiologists, who jumped almost eight percent to $211,000.

On the losing side were gastroenterologists and psychiatrists, who took a big dip—six and eight percent respectively, down to $206,000 for the former and only $110,000 for psychiatrists, a crisis that is creating a professional depression. Only G.P.s, who made $105,000 net, did more poorly. Other losers included ophthalmologists ($197,000) and neurosurgeons, who dropped four and five percent respectively.

But don't cry for the brain doctors—they netted the top dollar of $297,000 on a gross of almost a half million.

Still, the trend is to knock down high surgical prices, which had been going sky high. "I'll have clients in a surgical specialty," says a practice management consultant in Cincinnati, "tell me that their group's gross is down fifty thousand dollars per doctor." That is, except for heart surgeons, who are busier than ever and whose gross incomes rose fourteen percent to $427,000 each and are still rising.

It's important to understand that these numbers are *medians*, which mean that half the doctors earn more. By adding about twenty percent to the median salaries that we've described, we'll get the real figures for physicians practicing in large metropolitan areas.

Geography plays an important part in how well a doctor does. Surprisingly, doctors in the South—long pictured as a rural low-paying area—earn the most. The average gross in the South was $300,000, with a net of $169,000, reaching a peak in the Southwest, which includes booming Texas. There, the net was $175,100. Doctors in the East earned $10,000 to $15,000 less.

Medicare, on the other hand, pays according to the patient income levels in the area. More likely they will give a physician in Little Rock $27 for a simple office visit, as opposed to about $45 in Fairfield County, Connecticut, a New York City suburb, for the same work.

(We also have to consider whether doctors are not understating their net incomes. Thousands of them are audited by the IRS each year, with many having to pay large penalties for declaring less than they actually earned, or for taking excessive expenses from their relatively large grosses.)

Where the Big Money Is

We hear that some doctors make big money, and this is quite true at the upper levels of the practice. For example, the top 30 percent of heart surgeons have a net of over $400,000, while thirty-one percent of the top cardiologists—mainly in wealthy suburbs and cities—earned from $300,000 to $350,000. In fact, 15 percent of heart surgeons *netted* over $600,000, with no official report on how many hit the magic $1 million mark that doctors whisper about enviously.

Most of the big money is in surgery. The top 13 percent of neurosurgeons *netted $600,000 or more*, while 24 percent of orthopedists earned $350,000 to $400,000.

Just as the spread in income from doctor to doctor is large, so are the fees they charge their patients. A flexible sigmoidoscopy examination of the colon takes a median fee of $150, but the spread ranges from $75 to $275-plus. An injection for "Selective Coronary Angiography" can cost less than $150 and more than $800. The spread in fees among cardiologists for a "Left-heart Catheterization" is perhaps the largest, ranging from "less than $300" to over $2,000!

How is the patient to know? He can't, but he can seek out the best doctor he knows or can find through research, and worry about the money later—hoping much of it will be picked up by *some* third party.

Best Doctors Often Make the Least

In the money business of medicine, the people who try to practice best, and tend to be more idealistic, naturally make *less* money. Those are the academic physicians, whose incomes are quite reasonable but somewhat lower than those in private practice.

A recent report by the "Academic Practice Faculty Compensation and Production Survey, 1997" shows that pediatricians in the medical university system earn only

$102,553 (versus $129,000 in private practice), which rises to $120,000 for family practice doctors, to $155,300 for obstetrics/gynecology teachers, to $173,142 for ophthalmologists, to the ultimate, the man with the knife, the orthopedic surgeons, who take in $246,133—just $10,000 less than his private practice cousins.

These academic salaries are reasonable, and academic doctors can augment their income by taking on research grants, or by consulting for pharmaceutical companies by evaluating new drugs. But by and large, one does not get rich by teaching and researching at medical colleges.

Another study of doctors' incomes comes from the Medical Group Management Association, which includes 1,582 group practices. Their figures show incomes ranging from $125,000 for pediatricians, to $217,000 for obstetric/gynecology specialists, to $224,000 for gasatroenterologists, and $310,000 for orthopedic surgeons.

Of course, these are supposed *net* figures. The gross revenues of these practices are much higher. For example, internists took in $311,000, pediatricians $331,000, and orthopedic surgeons over $1 million.

Even the net figures are often understated in group practices, where many doctors receive a host of fringe benefits including retirement income payments, malpractice insurance, health insurance, among other factors—including a stake in the group's capitalization, which can mean a lot of money if they sell out or retire.

Working Harder to Keep Up the Mercedes

According to the Medical Group Management Association, primary doctors—family doctors, pediatricians, and internists—each had a patient roster of 2,000 in 1996, which in two years has grown to 2,300. The increased "productivity" keeps the doctor's income just as high, or higher than before, even though he may sometimes be getting lower fees.

The result, according to the doctor's own complaints,

is that in this HMO era, they are working harder, especially if they want to keep up their income. "Everyone is working harder," confirms a physician recruiter in Texas. He points out that family physicians who used see 26 to 28 patients a day, now see 30. Internists who used to see 15 to 20 patients a day, now see 22 to 26, with some handling 30.

The HMOs are having a strange effect on the field. Although doctors complain about low fees from some HMOs, they feel they *must* join up or be cut out of the future. *The dichotomy of the HMO-doctor love-hate relationship is that even though their fees are being discounted, the typical physician enrolled in an HMO (excluding the surgeons) is actually making more than his colleagues who eschew managed care.*

The reasons are many, including a flood of new patients on his roster, and capitation, where the doctor may get paid for five hundred patients up front, whether they get sick or not. One survey shows that doctors who participated in at least one HMO grossed $65,290 more than others who had no participation.

Years ago, doctors complained about low government compensation for Medicare patients on Part B (doctor's plan), and even threatened to boycott the aged. But in the new medical world, with lower payments from HMOs and even from indemnity insurers, Medicare checks are starting to look real good. Some doctors will take "Medicare Assignment," in which they agree to accept the Medicare schedule as their full compensation. The patient doesn't pay up front, and then pays only twenty percent of what Medicare allows the doctor.

But most doctors will not take "assignment." The doctor then can charge the Medicare patient 15 percent above the allowed amount. The patient pays the doctor up front, then waits perhaps six weeks for his reimbursement check. On a $100 bill from the doctor, for example, Medicare may allow about $85, and the patient must pay twenty percent of that, or $17 *plus* the $15 difference of $85 and $100. So in addition to his premiums of some

$550 a year, and a $100 deductible, the patient ends up paying thirty-two percent of the bill out-of-pocket.

New Fees—Most Are Higher

The Medicare compensation for doctors is being changed under the Balanced Budget plan of 1977, in which the government hopes to save money. But as of January 1, 1998, they have actually *raised* the pay of most physicians while cutting the amount going to surgeons. At the extremes, radiation oncologists, psychiatrists, radiologists, pathologists, and hematologists will get a substantial eight percent raise. Family and other primary doctors will get a six percent increase, while all surgeons will take a cut, up to almost nine percent for affluent heart surgeons.

In return, doctors will have to do even more paperwork than now. Medicare is issuing new guidelines—fifty-one pages worth—for the codes, which the doctors are supposed to document with each bill. In a Catch-22 situation, they are not *required* to fill out the heavy paper obligation. But if they don't, and they're audited, Medicare can deny the whole claim and penalize them besides. On the other hand, if they do the documentation, they will be safer when they upcode and ask for more money per visit.

Medicaid—The Bottom of the Medical Financial Barrel

Medicare has proven to be a blessing in disguise for doctors—especially as the patient population ages rapidly. But that's not true for the Medicaid program. The HHS pays doctors a meager amount per Medicaid visit, only two-thirds the Medicare allowance, or some $25 for a basic visit. It's too little for doctors to pay their bills, so most physicians just refuse to treat the poor in their offices.

What then do Medicaid patients do? Most use the emergency room of their local hospital as their "family doctor," a wasteful system. Just the "turnstile" at the E.R. has a hundred-dollar-plus tab, and with other charges, including the doctor's fee, a young, otherwise healthy child with a sore throat—perhaps seen by a nurse or a resident—will cost Medicaid several hundred dollars instead of the $35 for an office visit.

An attempt has been made to enroll Medicaid patients in HMOs to get them out of the expensive emergency rooms. About 30 percent of the poor have joined, some involuntarily. But there seems to be increasing resistance by HMOs to deal with the low government reimbursement. Recently, the Oxford plans—worried about their own survival—have announced that they are dropping Medicaid patients in Connecticut and New Jersey for not bringing in enough cash to pay for their cradle-to-grave care.

(There is a better way, which we'll explain in Chapter VIII, our plan for medicine in the twenty-first century.)

Physicians are always on the alert for increased revenue. One of the ways specialists do this is to concentrate on consulting, which pays considerably more than routine visits. This information comes from internal studies of doctors' practices, what one consultant calls "a statistical snapshot" that can add thousands of dollars a year to the doctor's bottom line.

This adviser points out that "it's best to have as many initial encounters [new patients] as possible qualify as consultations. Level by level, consults are paid at a higher rate than new—often 20 or 25 percent higher. These are dollars worth collecting." One doctor, an endocrinologist, accepts *only* patients who are referred to him by other doctors for "consultation."

Collect Every Last Dime

Another way to raise revenue, practice management people tell doctors, is to watch your collection ratio. A practice management expert tells of an internal medical practice that he thought was well-managed. "But I discovered that fifty percent of receivables were more than ninety days old." Also, insurance payments were lagging so badly that they represented almost one hundred percent of gross charges for a full year. (Many HMOs hold back money as long as they can to increase their cash flow and dampen that of doctors.)

The whole physician collection industry is highly organized. Where before, doctors excused bad debts after a few months, they now chase down the very last dollar by using collection agencies, who hound their patients and take about forty percent of the money collected themselves.

The Threat of Nurses

A new challenge to their pocketbook has now arisen in the form of nurse practitioners, who are being licensed in many states to do much of the work of primary physicians. The AMA has fought the concept from the beginning, but is losing the battle. Prior to 1998, these supernurses had to bill Medicare through an established doctor, which held them in check. But now they are on their own. As of January 1, 1998, nurse practitioners can bill Medicare directly for their services, at the reasonably high rate of eighty-five percent of the physician's fee schedule.

The whole concept of a nurse practitioner is somewhat illogical in the medical world, which claims there are too many doctors and that the number has to be cut down twenty percent. Meanwhile, the government—which, as we've seen—is paying New York hospitals a king's ransom *to train fewer physicians—is encouraging what is, in essence, thousands of new, less well trained doctors!*

Whatever is done to change the medical system, doctors will continue to earn enough to be near the top of economic heap. Their paranoia over the possible loss of their exaggerated incomes and their status in society is misplaced. In America today, doctors are and will remain godlike figures juggling life and death. However radically their profession is reformed, a doctor's money and his command of medical economics will no doubt be secure, and unfortunately, still uppermost in his mind.

Chapter VIII

A Plan for Tomorrow

How to Reform Medicine and Eliminate the Chaos

Americans have firmly rejected the single payer system of federal government medical care, what most call "socialized medicine," a system that exists in Britain and to some extent in our neighbor, Canada.

Americans fear—with good evidence in other areas to back them—that Washington will squander the money while depriving the intelligent patient of the freedom to choose his own pathway to health. This, of course, is what has happened in Britain, where a separate "private system" has evolved to make up for the logjam and inefficiencies of the government program.

Americans also fear that Washington will get dictatorial about their health care, controlling the number, description, and physical disposition of physicians and hospitals as part of a grand plan devised by theorists, one that offers goodies to the favored and poorer care to the majority, without any regard for the wishes of citizens of each community.

It is a sad commentary, but Americans do not trust Washington to be either efficient or fair. Especially with something as important as their health.

But despite their aversion to Washington, Americans must also admit that the so-called "free market" system is doing a miserable job of providing excellent medical care at a reasonable price. The reason is quite simple: there is no free market in medicine.

In no other area is the consumer (the patient) less able to gauge what is best for him, at the best price. Second, the so-called "free market" is more subject to professional monopoly than to competition.

Physicians Put Themselves First

Coming out of a medieval guild system, physicians have always put themselves first and the patient second despite the Hippocratic Oath. The doctor would like to help the patient, but not at the expense of his prime position of status and income. He would like to be free to follow his options, but is little concerned about the freedom of action of his patients.

The insurance companies, being almost all profit-making organizations, have almost nothing to do with medicine. They operate more like bookies, trying to figure the odds on how many people will get sick and how desperately, and how much it will cost them to insure that risk and still keep over 25 percent of the total (the "vigorish") for their inflated marketing and administrative expenses and profits—especially the obscene millions taken out of the medical pot by promoters who deny treatment to patients while they prosper.

Simultaneously, the insurers would like to shield themselves against the cost of severely sick patients who can cut into their profit margins. Their modus operandi is like that of a fire insurance company that will cover only small, less expensive homes.

Whether the care of Americans is controlled by insurance companies or physicians, or both, the consumer's best interests are generally the last concern in the priorities of this medical establishment. The result is medical chaos, one expressed in failed insurance and underinsurance, profits drained from medical costs, the excessive number of hospital beds, physician fraud, poorly trained doctors, a lack of uniform quality of care, the curtailing of needed care for the very sick, and numerous excesses and deficiencies in providing health care for us all.

In a way, this chaos isn't born of only a bad system. The tragic fact is that there is no cohesive system at all. It is one cobbled together from day to day, with no theory, no intelligent raison d'être. Chaos is truly the medical order of the day.

What then to do?

A New System Based on Patients

Washington is preparing a watered-down "Patient's Bill of Rights" to correct some of the problems raised by the ascendancy of the HMOs. But that is hardly the answer to the future of medicine in America.

The answer is to invent a whole new system that is indebted to neither Washington, the HMOs, the insurance industry, or the doctors. Instead, we need a methodology that puts patients first, last, and always.

Is it possible? I believe so, *if* the various special interest groups, including our politicians, would stop their selfish intransigence and false ideologies of left and right and start to concentrate on the American genius for civic good sense.

Who do Americans trust? Distant politicians? Absolutely not. But in every survey, the public has shown that it trusts itself and its local governments more than anyone else. In that local arena, close up, they have power—the ballot box, influence with friends and neighbors, the ability to speak out at town meetings, to write letters to the editors, to become active in community interest groups.

Loud voices that can move mountains locally are distant whispers in Washington. In the federal Beltway, those voices must be accompanied by lobbying power and money, something the typical voter lacks. Otherwise their voices will soon dissipate into that city's humid air.

Therefore, in an intelligent plan, good medical care must have a local base, one that equates the citizen and the patient as one and the same.

I have devised such a plan. I call it *Community Medicine.*

It is not designed as a pipe dream or a Utopian fantasy, but a plan that we can *start* to implement right now, one town at a time.

Let's take my own community, the lower southwest portion of Connecticut. In the twenty-five-mile stretch starting at the New York State border, there are some 500,000 people, which includes the affluent towns of Greenwich, Darien, New Canaan, Westport, and Weston.

But in any true Community Medical Plan (CMP), the population must be balanced. We cannot build a system based solely on the centers of affluence. In this case, balance there comes naturally because the area also includes the city of Bridgeport, one of the largest and poorest communities in the state.

The total 500,000 population of the district is an ideal size for community-based medicine. Not too small, nor too large to manage. Of the total, 142,000 of the citizens are in Bridgeport, where the minority population reaches 55 percent. In addition, the city of Stamford, which is closer to New York, has a population of 110,000, some 30 percent of whom are minorities. So, in many ways, the district is representative of America, both in its income and racial demographics.

How would a community health plan operate?

MAKING A COMMUNITY MEDICAL PLAN WORK

Here are the broad outlines of the plan. There would

be some five hundred in the nation and each would be an autonomous local group that is the umbrella for all medical activity in its area. It would be large enough to create efficiencies, yet small enough to learn if the reforms that are implemented are working, and how they can best be adjusted.

The CMP would have virtually full authority over the delivery of health care, including hospital usage and budget, medical insurance, physician activity and medical quality, and any fee setting that's necessary.

Most important, everyone who lives in the area would automatically be covered with medical insurance from the moment they are born. And each of the residents would have total freedom to see any physician in the area they wish, including specialists, and be a patient in any of the hospitals.

A medical board made up of physicians, hospital administrators, and individuals elected by the people of the area on a nonpolitical, independent basis would run an organization responsible for some $2 billion annually in cash, and for the health of all the occupants of the area.

What would they do? Virtually everything, starting with the hospitals in the area.

HOSPITAL OVERSIGHT

In this Connecticut area, as in almost all of America, the coordination between hospitals is virtually nil, something the CMP would deal with. Today, the quality of those institutions is only partially known, and only to the Joint Commission on hospital accreditation, whose measurements are uneven, insufficient, and poorly publicized. In this new arrangement, the CMP would be totally responsible for the evaluation—and enforcement, where necessary—of all hospitals in the area, for several factors including:

- Infection rate after surgery
- Ninety-day follow-up of infection rates, which are not now tallied

- Deaths and injuries in the hospital from iatrogenic, or doctor-caused, disease
- Adverse medication events and medication mistakes of inpatients and outpatients
- The amount of unnecessary surgery, by procedure—from tonsillectomy to open heart surgery
- The quality of surgery, with emphasis on errors

To accomplish this, the CMP would have a voluntary committee of physicians to oversee the quality, along with a full-time staff of evaluators. In the case of infections, a specialist in the area would set up guidelines to be followed. The federal CDC in Washington tries to *influence* hospitals on infections, apparently without success. But the CMP would have the *power* to enforce it.

In addition, the CMP would have the efficiency of scale in purchasing for all the hospitals, downsizing some and expanding others, trying to reduce the number of empty beds in the region.

HOSPITAL STAFF
The CMP Board would approve all hospital privileges and have a physician committee to recommend who shall be on staff, and who shall have those privileges taken away. This would be done by a regular audit by evaluators of physicians' work in the hospital and in the outpatient unit. Evaluation would involve not only reference to medical records, but random, on-site observation.

PHYSICIAN'S OFFICE QUALITY
One of the weakest links in quality care is what happens in the doctor's office, where *no one* has any idea of what kind of medicine the doctor is practicing. This must be changed. The CMP would set up a special auditing process carried out by a full-time staff of auditors and ethnographers, probably in conjunction with both a local law school and a medical college.

At least once every three years, *every* doctor practicing in the CMP area would be subject to an audit of his practice, a two-week process in which every patient's records would be examined, and some evaluation done on the spot. Other patients would be interviewed as to their experience with the doctor.

DOCTORS' CONTINUING EDUCATION

The CMP would do what the profession and the AMA has failed to do: set up a strict, *compulsory* continuing education program.

Each CMP in the nation would be attached to a university school of medicine. (Yale is just thirty miles from the center of the projected Southwestern Connecticut CMP.) Every doctor would become a student and/or teacher in the university, attending or teaching classes for at least one week a year full-time, plus twenty-five more hours of education a year *on site* at the college. The medical school would reward the best students with faculty, unpaid titles such as "Lecturer" or "Clinical Assistant Professor," up to "Clinical Professor."

Those who failed to complete their continuing education would be censured by the CMP. Continued failure would result in a recommendation from the CMP to the state for the suspension or revocation of the license to practice.

RECERTIFICATION OF THE LICENSE TO PRACTICE

Every seven years the CMP—under authorization from the state—would reexamine every doctor in the area on all aspects of medical care. Each physician would have three opportunities to pass the recertification examination, which will differ each time. If a doctor failed three times, his license to practice medicine would be suspended, then perhaps revoked after appeal.

OPEN RECORDS

The CMP would regularly publish for the public any negative information on doctors in the community, including suspension of hospital privileges, failure to keep up, Medicare "exclusion," and cases in which Medicare patients had complained of being overcharged, if the charges have been sustained by the government.

In the case of malpractice, the CMP would divulge the names and actions of doctors who have lost or settled three or more cases. In that event, the names of the physicians would be made public, along with a printed rebuttal by the doctors. No official action would be taken. It would be up to the patients to decide whether to patronize the doctors or not.

BOARD CERTIFICATION

All physicians enrolled with the CMP shall be required to be certified in at least one board of their choosing, including the three that cover primary care. They will receive three opportunities to pass their boards, plus an appeal. If they failed that, they would not be allowed to practice in the CMP, and recommendation would be made to the state to suspend, then perhaps to revoke their license to practice.

PREVENTIVE MEDICINE

Immunization of *all* residents would be undertaken by the CMP, including the necessary shots for children, and immunization of all adults for pneumococcus, hepatitis A, tetanus, and annual flu shots. Computer records for preventive care would be set up on all 500,000 residents, with notation of all immunizations given by the town health services, hospitals, and physicians. Notice would be sent out regularly to those who were not immunized, and doctors educated to educate their patients.

Preventive medicine is poorly practiced in America. The CMP would work with all physicians to improve the situation, including the following tests:

- Annual mammograms after fifty for women
- Pap smears on a regular basis
- Manual exams and blood tests for enlarged and possible cancerous prostates for men.

- Flexible sigmoidoscopy after age fifty to detect colon cancer
- Electrocardiogram exam every two years for patients over fifty

The results of these examinations would be entered on the patient's computer records, which would be available to all physicians in the community on a *confidential* basis.

AUTHORIZATION FOR CMP

The power exercised by the local CMP will be granted to it by the state, much as it now does for local school boards. In some cases, the CMP can operate independently once it has legal authorization from the state. In other situations, such as suspension of doctor liceneses, it would make recommendations to the state, and expect them to be carried out—minus extenuating circumstances or appeals that are sustained.

HEALTH INSURANCE FOR ALL

Everyone in the CMP would be insured from birth. Payment for this would be accomplished in many ways. The community would be helped by income from such federal programs as Medicaid, Public Health Service monies, and the new federal program that would insure needy children not on Medicaid.

The CMP would require that everyone in the community be insured—much as we now require insurance to drive a car. Those who do not have insurance would purchase it. If they cannot afford it and are not covered by Medicaid, the CMP and the state would pay. Part of this money would come from efficiencies in operation of community medicine.

WHO WILL PAY FOR THE MEDICAL CARE IN THE CMP?

As time goes by, the plan would be responsible for all medical expenditures in the community. Eventually, the CMP would pay all hospital bills, and those of doctors as well.

The CMP would receive the Medicaid money from the federal government and the state in bulk form, other federal monies for care of children, funds from HMOs in payment of care, and from the indemnity insurance companies. In addition, the CMP would collect from the patients the money now spent as co-payments on insurance, from whatever source.

The CMP would set fee schedules for all doctors in the area, equalizing the amount paid to doctors under Medicare and Medicaid. By properly compensating local doctors for Medicaid patients, they would eliminate the drain on hospitals in which the expensive emergency room is used by the poor as their "family doctor."

In addition, the CMP would save huge amounts by setting up pediatric clinics for children, eliminating the vast, current waste of Medicaid funds.

Monies that would normally go to the individual hospital or the individual doctor would instead go to the CMP, which would set a universal budget for all medical care in the area. This would enable the CMP to negotiate with the local hospitals on an overall yearly budget.

Similarly, the CMP would pay all the bills of doctors from the same general fund. A universal budget would be set up for all the doctors in the area. To ensure that they won't be "volumed" out by doctors attempting to practice more medicine to get more money, the computers would regulate the cash flow (as they now do in Germany) by paying only a proportionate amount from day one of the year in relation to the universal budget.

That would be done to ensure there would be money left in the till at the end of the year—unless the community was stung with a giant flu or other epidemic in December.

Each year, budgets with both the hospitals and the doctors in the area would be renegotiated, either up or down, depending on the year's experience.

WHAT ABOUT MEDICARE PATIENTS PRESENTLY WELL-INSURED?

Since the Medicare system for the aged is one of the best insurance systems in America—one that is sustained because of the political power of senior citizens—that would continue as is, without the aged patient having to be bound by CMP regulations.

However, the older patients would benefit enormously from CMP guidelines on quality care, preventive medicine, hospital standards, continuing education, discipline and recertification of physicians.

WHAT ABOUT MEDICAL CARE OUTSIDE THE CMP?

If the CMPs are well-designed, most patients will find every opportunity for quality care within the area, especially if it includes a medical college and university hospital, as it would in every case. In the sample Southwest Connecticut CMP, for example, patients would have the right to use the Yale–New Haven Hospital, which is attached to Yale School of Medicine. Even though it is not geographically contiguous to the district, it is close by, and would be the "learning center" and a major hospital for this and perhaps three more nearby CMPs.

However, should a local patient want to go outside the district for his care, he would be able to do that, at his wish, merely by paying a larger co-payment. Transfer of funds between CMPs for out-of-area care would be established.

CMPs AND THE HMOs

The CMP will help the local physicians in organizing against excesses of the HMOs by setting guidelines that *all* physicians in the community would have to follow. The HMOs, as well, would have to follow these CMP guidelines, or find that they cannot operate in that area.

Guidelines for the HMOs and other managed care insurance systems would include compulsory clauses in all contracts with local physicians that would prohibit the HMOs from having any medical power whatsoever.

The HMOs would have to give up their usual requirement of prior approval of treatment, which would be decided solely by local physicians. Consultation with specialists would be up to the patient, who would have unfettered access to any specialist in the CMP area. If so-called "experimental" techniques are available, it would be up to physicians to decide if the care was appropriate.

Most important, all capitation plans would be illegal. The physician would sign a pledge with the CMP that he will never enter into a contract with an insurance group to gain any financial advantage by reducing care to the patient.

THE POSSIBILITY OF PHASING OUT INSURANCE COMPANIES

The CMP, having 500,000 patients, might also eventually self-insure itself, much as some large corporations now do. In fact, that is the ideal situation because the overhead would be smaller, there would be no large marketing costs and no profit to be made.

This would mean the elimination of HMOs, and almost all insurance companies in America, except for the few that want to handle private insurance beyond the needs of CMP subscribers.

Until then, by having employers' contributions come directly to the CMP from companies where the subscribers work, maximum financial efficiency would be achieved.

No plan devised can be perfect, and surely there are suggestions that can be made to improve my Community Medicine system. But it is also obvious that Washington cannot achieve the goals of good, efficient medicine on the local level, and states are also generally too large to handle the problem. Only in the microcosm of the community is there the intimate knowledge, the common sense, the citizen participation from which can evolve better medicine for all.

There will be other solutions to the present chaos probably inferior to my plan, but there should be unanimous agreement that medicine as it is now practiced and delivered does not meet the needs of most Americans.

Faced with the challenge of shaping medical reform, I am convinced that the civic genius of America will conquer the day.

And the sooner the better.

Notes and Bibliography

Along with numerous personal interviews by the author, the following sources provided useful material for this book.

CHAPTER 1—THE HMO REVOLUTION

"Making Sense of Managed Care," John C. Rother, *Modern Maturity*, March/April 1997.

"What Managed Care Can't Seem to Manage Is Efficiency," Gary F. Kreiger, *American Medical News*, July 22, 1996.

"HMO Rules Will Expand Patient Rights and Create Arbitration Panel," Jennifer Preston, *New York Times*, February 5, 1997.

"Patients With Difficult Illnesses Fight New HMOs to Get Help," Elisabeth Rosenthal, *New York Times*, July 15, 1996.

"Choosing a Health Plan," Michelle G. Rapaport., *Consumers Digest*, May/June 1997.

"Tape Bares Renowned Cancer MD's Battle With Insurer," William Sherman, *New York Post*, September 21, 1995.

"They Cut Costs—Not Bosses' Pay," William Sherman, *New York Post*, September 22, 1995.

"Ex-New Yorker is Told: Get Castrated So We Can Save," William Sherman, *New York Post*, Septembr 18, 1995.

"Plan Nixed Vital Growth Drug For Teen," William Sherman, *New York Post*, September 19, 1995.

"How Low Can Fees Go?" Mark Crane, *Medical Economics*, April 7, 1997.

"Take My Freedom, Please. HMOs That Let You Choose Doctors Aren't the Right Choice," Ellyn E. Spragins, *Newsweek*, April 7, 1997.

"Can This Medical Plan Be Saved? How To Make Your Medical Plan-Work For You?" Peggy Moran, *Prevention*, April 1997.

"Is Your HMO OK—Or Not?" Janet Bryant Quinn, *Newsweek*, February 10, 1997.

"Ill Elderly and Poor Fare Worse in HMOs, Study Shows," David R. Olmos, *Los Angeles Times*, October 2, 1996.

"Quality of Care for Poor and Elderly at HMOs is Questioned in New Study," George Anders, *The Wall Street Journal*, October 2, 1996.

"Choosing an HMO," *Consumer Reports*, August, 1996.

"Rationed Health Care Serves the Bottom Line," Letter to the Editor, *New York Times*, July 21, 1996.

"How Doctors Can Regain Control of Health Care," Interview with Dr. Paul M. Elkwood, Jr., *Medical Economics*, May 13, 1996.

"Choosing an HMO," Daphna W. Gregg, *Harvard Health Letter*, April 1996.

"Choosing an HMO," Stuart Auerbach, *The Washington Post*, November 7, 1995.

"Beware Your HMO" (HMOs often delay or deny crucial care), Ellyn E. Spragins, *Newsweek*, October 23, 1996.

"Give Your HMO a Thorough Annual Checkup," Alan Mittermaier, *Wall Street Journal*, October 9, 1995.

"The Trouble with HMOs," M. Stanton Evans and Malcolm A. Kline, *Consumers' Research Magazine*, July 1995.

"What You Should Know About Your HMO—But Aren't Likely to Find Out," *Healthfacts*, July 1995.

"Prescription for Disaster," Michael E. DeBakey, Op-Ed column, *Wall Street Journal*, June 23, 1994.

"One Man's Battle With Managed Care," Betsy McCaughey Ross, Op-Ed column, *New York Times*, December 28, 1996.

"Trial May Put Managed Care to Test," Charles Ornstein, *Dallas Morning News*, December 15, 1997.

"Kaiser Agrees to Pay $5.35 Million in Death," Charles Ornstein, *Dallas Morning News*, December 17, 1997.

"When Care is Denied," *Los Angeles Times*, August 27, 1995.

"Don't Miss Out on Medicare Managed Care," Ken Terry, *Medical Economics*, April 7, 1997.

"The M.O. of Medicare HMOs," *Newsletter, People's Medical Society*, August 1995.

"A Mixed Diagnosis for HMOs," Michael A. Hiltzig and David R. Olmos, *Los Angeles Times*, August 27, 1995.

"State Widely Criticized for Regulation of HMOs," Michael A. Hiltzik and David R. Olmos, *Los Angeles Times*, August 28, 1995.

"Times Poll: Insured People Satisfied with Medical Care," Jim Schachter, *Los Angeles Times*, August 28, 1995.

"Family Prevails in Long Struggle with HMO," David R. Olmos and Michael A. Hiltzik, *Los Angeles Times*, August 28, 1995.

"Doctors' Authority, Pay Dwindle Under HMOs," David R. Olmos and Michael A. Hiltzik, *Los Angeles Times*, August 29, 1995.

"Specialists Finding Prognosis for Good Jobs is Grimmer," David R. Olmos, *Los Angeles Times*, August 29, 1995.

"Emergency Rooms, HMOs Clash Over Treatment and Payments," Michael A. Hiltzik, *Los Angeles Times*, August 30, 1995.

" 'Kaiser Justice' System's Fairness Is Questioned," Michael A. Hiltzik and David R. Olmos, *Los Angeles Times*, August 30, 1995.

"Are Executives at HMOs Paid Too Much Money?" Michael A. Hiltzik and David R. Olmos, *Los Angeles Times*, August 30, 1995.

"Pressure is Mounting for Better Oversight of HMOs," Michael A. Hiltzik and David R. Olmos, *Los Angeles Times*, August 31, 1995.

"San Diego in Lead of HMO Revolution," Barbara Marsh, *Los Angeles Times*, August 31, 1995.

"Gagging The Doctors," Paul Gray, *Time*, January 8, 1996.

"Can Managed Care Really Cut Health Care Costs?" Robert W. Stein, *Best's Review*, May 1995.

"Deadly Gag Rules," Peter L. Spencer, *Consumers' Research*, January, 1996.

"Beware The Secret Peril in HMOs," Steffie Woolhandler and Dvid U. Himmelstein, *Consumers' Research*, February 1996.

"How Your HMO Could Hurt You," *U.S. News and World Report*, January 15, 1996.

"Does Your HMO Stack Up?" Ellyn Spragins, *Newsweek*, June 24, 1996.

"Don't Let Them Rush You into an HMO," Bridgid McMenamin, Forbes, July 15, 1996.

"What To Know About Your HMO," *New York*, May 20, 1996.

"It Could Happen to You," Michael Parrish, *Health*, May/June 1996.

"Managed Care, Medicare: How To Make Them Work For You," *Modern Maturity*, November/December 1997.

"Three Big Health Plans Join in Calling For National Standards," Robert Pear, *New York Times*, September 25, 1997.

"Trend Toward Managed Care is Unpopular, Surveys Find," Peter T. Kilborn, *New York Times*, September 28, 1997.

"Panel of Experts Urges Broadening of Patient Rights," Robert Pear, *New York Times*, October 23, 1997.

"Health Maintenance Groups Are Seen Entering a Troublesome New Phase," Peter T. Kilborn, *New York Times*, November 22, 1997.

"Health Care at the Crossroads," (managed care), Arnold Birenbaum, *USA Today* (magazine), November 1997.

"A Bitter Pill for the HMOs," Milt Freudenheim, *New York Times*, April 28, 1995.

"How Good Is Your Health Plan?" *Consumer Reports*, August 1996.

"Prescription Switches," Bob Herbert, *New York Times*, December 27, 1996.

"What Is The Value of a Voice?" Linda Peeno, *U.S. News and World Report*, March 9, 1998.

"A Chance to Survive," Bob Herbert, *New York Times*, July 4, 1997.

"Doctors Organize to Fight Corporate Intrustion," Peter T. Kilborn, *New York Times*, July 1, 1997.

"Manage With Care," C. Everett Koop, *Time*, Special Issue, Fall, 1996.

"White House Adds Broad Protection in Medicare Rules," Robert Pear, *New York Times*, June 23, 1998.

"Panel Seeks HMO Overseer for California, a Bellwether," Todd S. Purdum, *New York Times*, January 6, 1998.

"HMO Premiums Rising Sharply, Stoking Debate on Managed Care," Ian Fisher, *New York Times*, January 11, 1998.

"Insurers Tighten Rules and Reduce Fees for Doctors," Milt Freudenheim, *New York Times*, June 28, 1998.

"Texas Allowing Suits Against HMO's," Sam Howe Verhovek, *New York Times*, June 5, 1996.

"Actuarial Firm Helps Decide Just How Long You Spend in Hospital," George Anders and Laurie McGinley, *Wall Street Journal*, June 15, 1998.

"A Medical Resistance Movement," Reed Abelson, *New York Times*, March 25, 1998.

"Rx for Reluctant Health Insurers," *Insight*, September 22, 1997.

"HMO Care Differs After Strokes," *New York Times* (AP), July 9, 1997.

"Health Insurers Skirting New Law, Officials Report," Robert Pear, *New York Times*, October 5, 1997.

"Medicare HMO's To Trim Benefits For the Elderly," Milt Freudenheim, *New York Times*, December 22, 1997.

"Largest HMOs Cutting the Poor and the Elderly," Peter T. Kilborn, *New York Times*, July 6, 1998.

"High Rates Hobble Law to Guarantee Health Insurance," Robert Pear, *New York Times*, March 17, 1998.

CHAPTER II—THE AMERICAN HOSPITAL

"Study Says Thousand Die From Reaction to Medicine," Denise Grady, *New York Times*, April 15, 1998.

The New Hands-Off Nursing," *Time*, September 30, 1996.

"An Alternative Strategy for Studying Adverse Events in Medical Care," Lori B. Andrews, et al., *The Lancet*, February 1, 1997.

"Our Ailing Public Hospitals: Cure Them or Close Them?" Jerome P. Kassirer, (Editorial), *The New England Journal of Medicine*, November 16, 1995.

"Public Advocate Says Hospital Accreditation System is Faulty," Ian Fisher, *New York Times*, January 21, 1998.

"Overview of Nosocomial Infections, Including the Role of the Microbiology Laboratory," T. Grace Emori and Robert P. Gaynes, *Clinical Microbiology Reviews*, October 1993.

"Effectiveness in Disease and Injury Prevention," *Morbidity and Mortality Weekly Report*, October 23, 1992.

"Incidence of Adverse Drug Events and Potential Adverse Drug Events: Implications for Prevention," David W. Bates et al., *JAMA*, July 5, 1995.

"Elite Cancer Center Gave Journalist Fatal Drug Dose," *Modern Healthcare*, March 27, 1995.

"Trends in Methicillin-Resistant Staphylococcus Aureus in United States Hospitals," Robert P. Gaynes, et al., *Infectious Diseases in Clinical Practice*, Volume 2, No. 6.

"Experts See Need to Control Antibiotics and Hospital Infections," Lawrence K. Altman, *New York Times*, March 12, 1998.

"Failure To Wash Up at Hospital Is Tied to Babies' Infection," *New York Times* (AP), March 13, 1997.

"Hospital Says It Shut Unit After 4 Babies Died," Philip Hilts, *New York Times*, September 16, 1997.

"Angioplasty in New York State, 1995," *New York State Department of Health,* Barbara A. DeBuono, Commissioner, Albany, New York.

"The Hazards of Hospitalization," Elihu M. Schimmel, *Annals of Internal Medicine,* January 1964.

"Nurses' Patient-Care Outlook Grim," J. Duncan Moore, Jr., *Modern Healthcare,* June 17, 1996.

"Hospitals Looking Abroad To Keep Their Beds Filled," Milt Freudenheim, *New York Times,* December 10, 1996.

"Quality of Care for Medicare Patients with Acute Myocardial Infarction," Edward F. Ellbeck, et al, *JAMA,* May 17, 1995.

"L.I. Debates Future of Its Empty Hospital" (psychiatric), *New York Times,* November 5, 1996.

"Measuring Quality, Improving Performance," *The Joint Commission on Accreditation of Healthcare Organizations,* Oakbook Terrace, Illinois.

"Are Hospitals Headed for Intensive Care?" Paul Wallich, *Scientific American,* April 1994.

"Hospitals Aren't Candid on Poor Care, a Study Says," Ian Fisher, *New York Times,* April 1, 1998.

"Hospitals Profit on Medicare," Julie Johnsson, *American Medical News,* January 8, 1996.

"A Delicate Balancing Act" (sale of non-profit hospitals to for-profits), Jay Greene, *Modern Healthcare,* March 13, 1995.

"Data Driving Quality Advance: But Outcome Numbers May Leave Consumers in the Dark," Linda Oberman, *American Medical News,* January 17, 1994.

"The Prescription That Kills" (reducing medication errors in hospitals), Geoffrey Cowley, *Newsweek,* July 17, 1995.

"Lack of Oversight Takes Delivery-Room Toll," Jane Fritsch and Dean Baquet, *New York Times,* March 6, 1995.

"More For-Profit Chains Court Public Hospitals," Sandy Lutz, *Modern Healthcare,* May 15, 1995.

"Columbia/HCA Planning to Cut Network by at Least a Third," Kurt Eichenwald, *New York Times,* November 17, 1997.

"Hospitals Overwork Novice Doctors and Leave Them Unsupervised," *New York Times*, December 14, 1997.

"Coronary Artery Bypass Surgery in New York State, 1993–1995," *New York State Department of Health*, Albany, New York, August 1997.

"Hospital Gets Fine on Hours Young Doctors Have to Work," Ian Fisher, *New York Times*, June 16, 1998.

"Fat's In The Fire Over Hospitals' Illegal Ops," Greeg Birnbaum and Jackie Rothenberg, *New York Post*, December 19, 1997.

"2 Hospitals Fined In Wake of Death of 'Rent' Creator," Elisabeth Rosenthal, *New York Times*, December 13, 1996.

"Twelve New York Hospitals Receive Surprise Visits From State Inspectors," Esther B. Fein, *New York Times*, March 12, 1998.

"Study: Many Elderly Given Wrong Drugs," Peter Eisler, *USA Today*, November 17, 1997.

"Hospital Characteristics and Quality of Care," Emmett B. Keeler, et al, *JAMA* October 7, 1992.

"Nurses Get New Role in Patient Protection: Pact With Biggest HMO Allows Care Givers to Guard Standards," Peter T. Kilborn, *New York Times*, March 26, 1998.

"Study Finds Drug-Reaction Toll Is High," *Wall Street Journal*, April 15, 1998.

CHAPTER III—THE EPIDEMIC OF MEDICAL THIEVERY

Semiannual Reports, Office of Inspector General, Department of Health and Human Services, October 1, 1994 through March 31, 1997 (six volumes), June Gibbs Brown, Inspector General.

Statement of George F. Grob, Deputy Inspector General, HHS, before the Senate Committee on Labor, HHS, and Education, October 2, 1995.

"Patient Abuse and Neglect: The Hidden Crime," *National Association of Medicaid Fraud Control Units*, May, 1997.

Testimony of Michael Mangano, Principal Deputy Inspector General, HHS, before the House Budget Committee, April 4, 1995.

Testimony of June Gibbs Brown, Inspector General, HHS, before the

House Subcommittee on Human Resources and Intergovernmental Relations, March 22, 1995.

Statement of June Gibbs Brown, Inspector General, HHS, before the House Subcommittee on Labor, HHS and Education, January 12, 1995.

"Annual Report, State Medicaid Control Units," *Office of Inspector General*, HHS, March 1997.

"Exclusions From Medicaid and Other Federal Health Care Programs," hearing before the House Subcommittee on Human Resources and Intergovernmental Affairs, September 4, 1996.

"Medicaid Fraud Report," *National Association of Attorneys General*, July/August 1996.

"Medicaid Fraud Report," *National Association of Attorneys General*, June 1997.

"Medicare Fraud and Abuse," testimony of Albert A. Hallmark, Regional Inspector General, HHS, April 11, 1994.

Statement by Michael Mangano, Principal Deputy Inspector General, HHS, before the House Subcommittee on Health.

"Health Care Fraud Program," *Criminal Investigative Division, Federal Bureau of Investigation.*

"Feds Come Knocking in Search of Home-Care Fraud," John Burns, *Modern Healthcare*, June 5, 1995.

"Wide Raids Made on Hospital Chain: U.S. Focuses on Expenses That Columbia/HCA Units Filed," Kurt Eichenwalk, *New York Times*, July 17, 1997.

"Audit of Medicare Finds $23 Billion in Overpayments," Robert Pear, *New York Times*, July 17, 1997.

"A Gold Mine in False Claims," Julie Johnsson, *American Medical News*, October 28, 1996.

"Medical Charges Settled; Hospitals Say Claims Were Made on Advice of Consultants," *Modern Healthcare*, May 12, 1997.

"Five Doctors Indicted in Medicare Home Care Scam," *American Medical News*, September 1, 1997.

"U.S. Indicts 12 in $15 Million Medicare Ring," *New York Times*, August 8, 1997.

"Visionary Resigns Under Scrutiny" (Columbia/HCA Healthcare), *U.S. News and World Report*, August 4, 1997.

"Preventing and Controlling Health Insurance Fraud," *Health Insurance Association of America*, Washington, D.C., January 1991.

"What HHS' War on Fraud and Abuse Means to You," Michael Pretzer, *Medical Economics*, August 25, 1997.

"Bad Practices" (Federal probe of Columbia/HCA), Michael Hirsh and Daniel Klaidman, *Newsweek*, August 11, 1997.

"Guess Who's in the Waiting Room" (The Feds widen their crackdown of Medicare overbilling), Susan B. Garland, *Business Week*, August 11, 1997.

"Is Fraud Poisoning Home Health Care," *Business Week*, March 14, 1994.

"Federal Judge Upholds $1 Billion Medicare Fraud Lawsuit Against Allina Hospitals," (Nurse Anesthetists vs. Anesthesiologist), *PR Newswire*, September 30, 1997.

"Columbia Inquiry Yields First Indictment," Eva M. Rodriguez and Lucette Lagnado, *Wall Street Journal*, July 31, 1997.

"3 Executives of Hospital Chain Charged With Medicare Fraud," Kurt Eichenwald, *New York Times*, July 31, 1997.

"Hospital Chain Cheated U.S. On Expenses, Documents Show," Kurt Eichenwald, *New York Times*, December 18, 1997.

"Ga. Home-Care Firm Convicted of Fraud (ABC Home Health Services), *Modern Healthcare*, February 12, 1996.

"Audits Target Teaching Doc's Claims," Karen Pallarito, *Modern Healthcare*, September 23, 1996.

"Lab Firms Fined Record $187 Million for Medicare Fraud," Julie Johnsson, *American Medical News*, December 9, 1996.

"Diagnose and Excise Fraud in Medicare," Michael Bilirakis, *Insight*, June 19, 1995.

"The High Cost of Fraud: Consumers in an Ideal Spot to Catch Medicare Cheats," Annette Winter, *Modern Maturity*, March-April 1997.

"Columbia/HCA Blood Test Bills Probed," Greg Jaffe and George Anders, *Wall Street Journal*, July 23, 1997.

"NME to Pay Fine of $379 Million," Sandy Lutz, *Modern Healthcare*, July 4, 1994.

"Hospitals face a U.S. Inquiry in Newark," (FBI Investigation), Ronald Smathers, *New York Times*, June 23, 1997.

"83 Massachusetts Hospitals Make Feds' List," Donald Burda, *Modern Healthcare*, May 27, 1996.

"Story of Jack Mills Is Lesson in the Difficulty of Policing Medicare," George Anders, *Wall Street Journal*, July 21, 1997.

"Operation Restore Trust Nabs Physicians for Fraud," Eric Freedman, *American Medical News*, June 17, 1996.

"Is Medical Abuse an Epidemic?" *Business Week*, September 22, 1997.

"RX for the Black Market" (Medicaid pharmaceutical exposé), Douglas Kennedy, *New York Post*, April 19, 1995.

"Two Indicted in Medicare Fraud Probe," Angela Gonzalez, *The Business Journal* (Phoenix, Arizona), July 28, 1995.

"Fraud and Waste in Medicare," Editorial, *New York Times*, August 1, 1997.

"U.S. Auditing Five Hospitals In New York: Part of a National Effort to Stop Medicare Fraud," Esther B. Fein, *New York Times*, April 5, 1998.

"Piercing Medicare's Shadows: Public Policy Detective Malcolm Sparrow Draws Surprising Conclusions About Fraud," Leah K. Glasheen, *AARP Bulletin*, October 1997.

CHAPTER IV—MEDICAL INCOMPETENCE

"Quality of Health Care, Part 2: Measuring Quality of Care," Robert H. Brook, et al., *New England Journal of Medicine*, September 26, 1996.

"Practice Guidelines: To Be Or Not To Be," Robert H. Brook, *The Lancet*, October 12, 1996.

"Does Inappropriate Use Explain Geographic Variations in the Use of Health Care Services?" Mark R. Chassin, *JAMA*, November 13, 1987.

"Quality of Care: Time to Act," Mark R. Chassin, *JAMA* (Editorial), December 25, 1991.

"Impact of Quality-of-Care Factors on Pediatric Intensive Care Unit Mortality," Murray M. Pollack, et al., *JAMA*, September 28, 1994.

"Quality of Care, Process, and Outcomes In Elderly Patients With Pneumonia," Thomas P. Meehan, et al., *JAMA*, December 17, 1997.

"Variation in Office-Based Quality: A Claims-Based Profile of Care Provided to Medicare Patients with Diabetes," Jonathan P. Weiner, *JAMA*, May 17, 1995.

"Quality Health Care," Linda A. Headrick and Duncan Neuhauser, *JAMA*, June 7, 1995.

"Assessing Strategies for Quality Improvement," Mark R. Chassin, *Health Affairs*, May/June 1997.

"Getting The Best," *Harvard Health Letter*, January 1995.

"AMA Accrediation to Be Lean on Specifics," *Modern Healthcare*, May 26, 1997.

"Who's On First? The Primary Care Provider," *Newsletter-People's Medical Society*, April 1994.

"AMA Panel on Guidelines Sorts Good From Misguided," Linda Oberman, *American Medical News*, January 10, 1994.

"AMA Gets OK for Accreditation, Guidelines Projects," Linda O. Prager, *American Medical News*, December 23, 1996.

"AMAP-standard Setting for Physicians, by Physicians," Gary F. Krieger, *American Medical News*, January 20, 1997.

"Underuse of Coronary Revascularization Procedures," Marianne Laouri, *Journal of the American College of Cardiology*, April 1997.

"Changes to National Practitioner Data Bank Reporting—Effective or Not?" David E. Manoogian, *Physician Executive*, July 1944.

"Needed: A More Practical Way to Establish and Maintain Quality Control" (American Medical Accrediation Program), *American Medical Association*, Chicago, Illinois, 1997.

"Doctors Urged to Admit Mistakes," Denise Grady, *New York Times*, December 9, 1997.

"Benefit of Independent Double Reading in a Population-based Mammography Screening Program," Erik L. Thurfjell, et al., *Radiology*, April 1994.

"Variability in Radiologists' Interpretation of Mammograms," Joanna G. Elmore, et al., *New England Journal of Medicine*, December 1, 1994.

"The Accuracy of Mammographic Interpretation" (Editorial), *New England Journal of Medicine*, December 1, 1994.

"Risk of False Alarms from Mammogram is 50% Over Decade," *New York Times* (AP), April 15, 1998.

"More Lab Mistakes in Doctors' Offices," *New York Times* (AP), February 11, 1997.

"Quality of Care for Medicare Patients With Acute Myocardial Infarction," Edward F. Ellerbeck, et al., *JAMA*, May 17, 1995.

"Listening to the Heart; Dying Art?" Denise Grady, *New York Times*, September 3, 1997.

"Heart Care: New Doubts About an Old Test" (Report on a *JAMA* study), *U.A. News and World Report*, September 30, 1996.

"The Code of Silence," Gina Bradley, R.N. (a pseudonym with Kathryn Casey, *Ladies' Home Journal*, June 1997.

"In New Jersey, AMA Unveils National Test to Grade Doctors," Jennifer Preston, *New York Times*, November 19, 1997.

"Naked Before The World: Will Your Medical Secrets Be Safe in the New National Databank?" Ellyn E. Spragins and Mary Hager, *Newsweek*, June 30, 1997.

"16,638 Questionable Doctors: Disciplined by States or the Federal Government," Sidney Wolfe, et al., *A Public Citizen Health Research Report*, 1998.

"Focusing on Quality in a Changing Health System," *National Academy of Sciences*.

"Relation Between Surgeons' Practice Volume and Geographic Variation in the Rate of Carotid Endartrerectomy," Lucian L. Leape, et al., *New England Journal of Medicine*, September 7, 1989.

"Physician Profile," *Massachusetts Board of Registration in Medicine*, Boston, Mass., 1998.

"Checking Up on Your Doctor: What You Can Find Out." *Consumer Reports*, November 1996.

"How Does Your Practice Compare?" (Peer Review Organization pilot project), Linda Oberman, *American Medical News*, August 1, 1994.

"Medical Errors Bring Calls for Change," Lawrence K. Altman, *New York Times*, July 18, 1995.

"When Diagnosis Is Dire, Right Doctor Is the Key" (Case of Gregory White Smith), *USA Today*, October 6, 1997.

"Quality of Measurement or Quality of Medicine?" (Editorial), David B. Nash, *JAMA*, May 17, 1995.

"Visit Vegas! Get Your Boards While You're There," Ken Terry, *Medical Economics*, February 13, 1995.

"State Medical Boards Discipline More, Want Role in Health System Reform," Charles Marwick, *JAMA*, June 8, 1994.

"Should the Public Have Access to the National Practitioner Data Bank?" Jim Montague, *Hospitals and Health Networks*, June 5, 1994.

"New Anesthesia Rules" (Hazards of office anesthesia use), *American Medical News*, September 12, 1994.

"Variation in the Use of Medical and Surgical Services By the Medicare Population," Mark R. Chassin, et al., *New England Journal of Medicine*, January 30, 1986.

CHAPTER V—UNNECESSARY SURGERY

"Hysterectomy: Overused or Appropriately Performed?" Barbara Apgar, *American Family Physician*, February 15, 1997.

"Hysterectomy, Indications, Alternatives and Predictors," Marcia G. Kramer and Robert C. Reiter, *American Family Physician*, February 15, 1997.

"Unnecessry Hysterectomy: The Controversy That Will Not Die," *HealthFacts*, July 1993.

"The Appropriateness of Hysterectomy," Steven J. Bernstein, et al., *JAMA*, May 12, 1993.

"Hysterectomy and Its Alternatives," *HealthFacts*, May 1994.

"Study Tracks Hysterectomies. (Unnecessary surgery can be prevented through patient advocacy). *Cancer Research Weekly*, November 7, 1994.

"50,000 Unnecessary Appendectomies A Year—and How to Prevent Them," Edwin W. Brown, *Medical Update*, February 1997.

"Just Say No: Test Reduced Need for Appendix Removal," Yun lee Wolfe, *Prevention*. April 1997.

"Tonsil and Adenoid Surgery," *Clinical Reference Systems*, December 1994.

"Is the Treatment Really Working?", *The Guardian*, July 15, 1997.

"Cut Or Run?" Richard Laliberte, *Men's Health*, May 1995.

"When Less is More in Coronary Care," Mike McNamee, *Business Week*, October 3, 1994.

"The Endangered Gallbladder," *Consumer Reports on Health*, September 1995.

"Is That Operation Really Necessary?" Marvin M. Lipman, *Consumer Reports on Health*, April 1996.

"Questions To Ask Your Doctor Before You Have Surgery," *Executive Health's Good Health Report*, May 1996.

"The Appropriateness of Carotid Endarterectomy," Constance M. Winslow, et al., *New England Journal of Medicine*, March 24, 1988.

"Carotid Endarterectomy for Elderly Patients: Predicting Complications," Robert H. Brook, et al., *Annual of Internal Medicine*, November, 1990.

"Predicting the Appropriate Use of Carotid Endarterectomy, Upper Gastrointestinal Endoscopy, and Coronary Angiography," *New England Journal of Medicine*, October 25, 1990.

"Surgery to Prevent Stroke May Cause It, Study Shows," *New York Times* (AP), February 6, 1998.

"Adopting Practice Patterns to a Managed Care Environment: Carotid Endarterectomy—A Case Example," Robert H. Brook, *Journal of Vascular Surgery*, May 1996.

"Some Hospitals Found to Cash-In on C-Sections," Evelyn Gilbert, *National Underwriter Property & Casualty-Risk and Benefits Management*, February 4, 1991.

"Health Care's Weird Geography" (editorial), *New York Times*, October 25, 1997.

"An Unkind Cut," Paula Dranov, *American Health*, September 1990.

"Is This Operation Really Necessary?" Steve Salerno, *The American Legion*, April 1993.

"Alternative Strategies for Controlling Rising Cesarean Section Rates," Randall S. Stafford, *JAMA*, February 2, 1990.

"Unnecessary Cesarean Sections: Curing a National Epidemic," Sidney M. Wolfe, Mary Gabay, *Public Citizen's Health Research Group*, May 1994.

"A Landmark Verdict on an Unnecessary Cesarean," Vicki Elson, *Special Delivery*, Spring 1994.

"Consumer Group Challenges C-Section Rate" (Public Citizen), *Special Delivery*, Summer 1994. Reprinted from *Ann Arbor News*, May 19, 1994.

"Does Inappropriate Use Explain Small-Area Variations in the Use of Health Care Services?" Lucian L. Leape, et al., *JAMA*, February 2, 1990.

"An International Comparison of Back Surgery Rates," Daniel C. Cherkin, Richard A. Deyo, et al., *SPINE*, Volume 19, Number 11, 1994.

"Low Back Pain Hospitalization, Recent United States Trends and Regional Variations," Victoria M. Taylor, Richard A. Deyo, et al., *SPINE*, Volume 19, Number 11, 1994.

"Federal Agency Under Fire; Finds Most Back Surgery Unnecessary," *HealthFacts*, October 1995.

"Neurosurgeon Criticizes Spine Surgeons," *The Back Letter*, February, 1994.

"Study Sees Overuse of Ear Operation," Jane E. Brody, *New York Times*, April 27, 1994.

"The Medical Appropriateness of Tympanostomy Tubes Proposed For Children Younger Than 16 Years in the United States," Lawrence C. Kleinman, et al., *JAMA*, April 27, 1994.

CHAPTER VI—THE MAKING OF A MODERN DOCTOR

"More Geriatric Training Needed as Population Ages," Deborah Shelton, *American Medical News*, November 11, 1996.

"Educational Programs in U.S. Medical Schools, 1995–1996," Barbara Barzansky, et al., *JAMA*, September 4, 1996.

"The Changing Face of American Medical Education," Myles N. Sheehan, *America*, February 10, 1996.

"Freezing The Number of Residency Positions," (Letter to the Editor and reply), Robert G. Luke and Kenneth I. Shine, *JAMA*, September 6, 1995.

"Student Program Spurs Generalism At Medical Schools," Jim Montague, *Hospitals and Health Networks*, April 20, 1994.

"Behind The White Coat," Alan Bonsteel, *The Humanist*, March/April 1997.

"Peformance on the National Board of Medical Examiners; Part I, Examination By Men and Women of Different Race and Ethnicity," Beth Dawson, et al., *JAMA*, September 4, 1994.

"Minority Students in Medical Education: Facts and Figures IX, *Association of American Medical Colleges*, Winter 1996.

"Medical Education in the United States and Canada," Carnegie Foundation for the Advancement of Teaching, 1910. Reprinted by *Science and Health Publications*, 1960.

"Educational Programs in U.S. Medical Schools," (Figures on student academic failures), Barbara Barzansky, et al., *JAMA*, September 6, 1995.

"1000 Hospitals Will Be Paid to Reduce Supply of Doctors," Warren E. Leary, *New York Times*, August 25, 1997.

"Are We Choosing The Best Students for Medical School?" Gary F. Krieger, *American Medical News*, October 3, 1994.

"Accreditor Proposes Tighter Rein on Residency Programs," Leigh Page, *American Medical News*, March 27, 1995.

"Cheating on M.D. Test," *New York Times* (AP), August 2, 1997.

"The Doctor Glut: Experts Debate Predictions of a Physician Surplus," *Scientific American*, February, 1996.

"Let The Market For Doctors Heal Itself," Keith H. Hammonds, *Business Week*, March 10, 1997.

"Bulletin of Information, United States Medical Licensing Examination," *USMLE Secretariat*, Philadelphia, Pa.

"Doctor Ranks Grow 17 percent in Five Years," Mike Mitka, *American Medical News*, February 3, 1997.

"Getting The Scoop on Your Doctor," *Tufts University Health and Nutrition Letter*, March 1997.

"Is Residency Training Really Harmful?" (Letter to the Editor, plus reply.), John R. DeQuardo and Charles Rainey, *JAMA*, July 2, 1997.

"Graduate Medical Education and Government Oversight," Letter questioning "surplus" of doctors, plus reply, Lee Balaklaw, et al, *JAMA*, November 19, 1997.

"Shut Schools or Cut Students? Pew Commission Report Revives Debate on Physician Supply?" Mike Mitka, *American Medical News*, December 11, 1995.

"Medicare Funding for Medical Education: A Waste of Money?" Scott Gottlieb, *USA Today* (Magazine), November 1997.

"Teaching Hospitals Warn Shift to Primary Care May Hurt Specialist Programs" Bruce Japsen and Sandy Lutz," *Modern Healthcare*, April 3, 1995.

"B. E. Begone" (discontinuance of "board eligible" designation), *Newsletter-People's Medical Society*, August 1997.

"Expanding Generalist Work Force Seen As Ill-Conceived," *American Medical News*, September 11, 1995.

"Bridging the Gap Between Research and Practice; The Role of Continuing Education," William Campbell, et al, *JAMA*, January 8, 1997.

"JAMA Now Will Offer CME (Continuing Medical Education) for Journal Reading," Mike Mitka, *American Medical News*, November 10, 1997.

CHAPTER VII—MEDICAL ECONOMICS AND THE AMERICAN DOCTOR

"Physicians Heal Themselves," Lawrence A. Kudlow and Steve Moore, *National Review*, September 26, 1994.

"In Congress, Haste Makes More Than Waste," Aaron Epstein, *Knight-Ridder/Tribune News Service*, August 9, 1994.

"Member Services: Profiles of Management Service and Physician Management Companies," *American Medical News*, November 25, 1996.

"Economics: Physicians' Incomes for Set-Fee Structures," John M. Eisenberg, *JAMA*, June 1, 1994.

"You Can Be an Eight-Minute Marcus Welby," Susan Harrington Preston, *Medical Economics,* October 13, 1997.

"Providers Should Weigh Risks of Risk Assumption," Clark W. Bell, *Modern Healthcare,* January 29, 1996.

Figures on doctors incomes, in general, and by specialty, from the AMA and Medical Economics Continuing Survey and other sources.

"Total Health Care Spending in '95 Was Nearly $1 Trillion," *National Underwriter Life and Health—Financial Services Edition,* February 10, 1997.

"Get the Highest Coding You're Entitled To," Anne L. Finger, *Medical Economics,* August 25, 1997.

"Economics: Physicians Incomes and Set-Fee Structures," John M. Eisenberg, *JAMA,* June 1, 1994.

"Profiles of Management Services and Physician Management Companies," *American Medical News,* November 25, 1996.

"What You Can Earn in a Large Group, Wayne J. Guglielmo, *Medical Economics,* March 25, 1996.

"Medical Bill Reviews Can Save Big Money," Brian Christine, *Risk Management,* October 1994.

"The Journal's Policy on Cost-Effectiveness Analyses," Editorial, *New England Journal of Medicine,* September 8, 1994.

"Profitable Capitation Requires Accurate Costing," David A. West, et al, *Nursing Economics,* May/June 1996.

"Economics" (Contempo), Uwe E. Reinhardt, *JAMA,* June 19, 1996.

"Providers Should Weigh Risks of Risk Assumption," Clark W. Bell, *Modern Healthcare,* January 29, 1996.

CHAPTER VIII—A PLAN FOR TOMORROW

This chapter draws on all the information of the previous chapters.

Index

About the Author

Martin L. Gross has established a nationwide reputation as an outspoken social critic. He has written a series of nonfiction political critiques, three of which have become *New York Times* best-sellers.

His first, *The Government Racket: Washington Waste from A to Z*, reached number three on the *Times* list and triggered a widespread debate on government spending and the need for reform. He has testified before the U.S. Congress five times, and has received praise from both sides of the aisle and from the White House. His other best-sellers are *A Call for Revolution: How Washington Is Strangling America*, and *The Tax Racket*.

Most recently, Mr. Gross wrote *The End of Sanity: Social and Cultural Madness in America*, which stimulated a continuing debate on national mores.

In the field of medicine, *The Doctors*, his first critique

of the profession, and the forerunner of *The Medical Racket*, was a huge success in 1967, resulting in several reforms in the way medicine was practiced.

His other books include *The Political Racket, The Brain Watchers,* and *The Psychological Society*—critiques of the political establishment, academic testing, and psychology and psychiatry, respectively—all of which aroused considerable controversy within these professions, and stimulated Congressional hearings and reform.

Mr. Gross has appeared on numerous national television programs across America, including "Larry King Live," "20/20," "Good Morning America," "Prime Time Live," and "CBS This Morning," as well as on CNN, the Fox News Network, PBS, and C-Span. The former editor-in-chief of *Book Digest,* he is an experienced Washington reporter whose syndicated column, "The Social Critic," appeared in newspapers throughout the country, from the *Los Angeles Times* to the *Chicago Sun-Times* to *Newsday*.

Mr. Gross has served on the faculty of the New School for Social Research and has been Adjunct Associate Professor of Social Science at New York University. He lives and works in Connecticut.